To Laura

Best Regards

[signature]

May-4th-2019

MIND
MEDICINE

Use Your Thoughts to Heal

DR. MAHMOUD RASHIDI, MD, FRCSC, FACS

The Brain Surgeon Who Had Brain Surgery

BALBOA
PRESS

A DIVISION OF HAY HOUSE

This book is a work of non-fiction. Unless otherwise noted, the author and the publisher
make no explicit guarantees as to the accuracy of the information contained in this book
and in some cases, names of people and places have been altered to protect their privacy.

Balboa Press books may be ordered through booksellers or by contacting:

Balboa Press
A Division of Hay House
1663 Liberty Drive
Bloomington, IN 47403
www.balboapress.com
1 (877) 407-4847

Because of the dynamic nature of the Internet, any web addresses or links contained in
this book may have changed since publication and may no longer be valid. The views
expressed in this work are solely those of the author and do not necessarily reflect the
views of the publisher, and the publisher hereby disclaims any responsibility for them.

The author of this book does not dispense medical advice or prescribe the use
of any technique as a form of treatment for physical, emotional, or medical
problems without the advice of a physician, either directly or indirectly. The
intent of the author is only to offer information of a general nature to help you
in your quest for emotional and spiritual well-being. In the event you use any
of the information in this book for yourself, which is your constitutional right,
the author and the publisher assume no responsibility for your actions.

Any people depicted in stock imagery provided by Getty Images are
models, and such images are being used for illustrative purposes only.
Certain stock imagery © Getty Images.

Print information available on the last page.

ISBN: 978-1-9822-0447-1 (sc)
ISBN: 978-1-9822-0449-5 (hc)
ISBN: 978-1-9822-0448-8 (e)

Library of Congress Control Number: 2018905999

Balboa Press rev. date: 08/10/2018

Dedication

For my kind, loving, and hardworking
parents; I love you very much.

Acknowledgments

I am very grateful to:

- My family for their unconditional love and acceptance of what I do and their support,

- Steve Harrison's Quantum Leap team for their help,

- My patients, from whom I learned so much,

- All my teachers and mentors, to whom I will always be indebted,

- And, of course, Ann McIndoo, my Author's Coach, who got this book out of my head and into my hands.

Contents

Introduction

I have written *Mind Medicine: Use Your Thoughts to Heal* because of my interest in the brain, thoughts, happiness, health, healing, and my own personal and professional life experiences. I care deeply about people's happiness, health, and healing. I have had the desire to help others be happy and healthy since my childhood. All my life, I have been interested in the mind and brain, their functions, and their effects on our lives.

I studied neurosurgery at the University of Toronto, Canada. I became sick and had surgery during my neurosurgery residency in Canada. Fortunately, I recovered and graduated, going to a fellowship in pediatric neurosurgery. During this period, I was very positive and never had doubts that I would heal. I have been practicing academic and private neurosurgery in the United States for more than sixteen years. I have treated thousands of adult and pediatric neurosurgical patients. These patients had different problems, from back pain to trauma and brain tumors.

During my neurosurgery practice, I noticed that happy and positive patients healed faster and returned to daily life quicker than unhappy and negative patients. When I researched this phenomenon, I found that it has been shown in multiple studies that our attitude affects our health and healing. This realization inspired me to write this book for people who are suffering from physical or emotional illness. People with depression, anxiety, worries, and stress will benefit from this book. I will teach them how to use their thoughts to help themselves heal. This book helps patients who are recovering from any illness, because it teaches them what to think and focus on while they are in the process of healing. As they are getting the proper medical and surgical treatment, they need to follow a positive and optimistic thought process which not only affects their body healing, but also gives them energy and stamina to persist and not quit.

I start this book by talking about my own story, which I hope to give the reader the confidence and hope that we all can heal. The healing starts from ourselves, not waiting for somebody to heal us.

Then I talk about the brain. Everything that I ask you to do from positive thinking and happiness, to optimism and hope, and to peaceful mind, all take place in your own brain. When you know more about the structure and function of your brain and become aware that your brain does all these functions, it will make more sense to you that You can control and use your brain in such ways. You want to control your thoughts in your own brain. You are not trying to control something outside you. Remember, it is your brain and you can use it the way you want. It may be uncomfortable for some people when I suggest that your mind is the result of your brain function but, based on my experience and observation of many patients as well as neuroscience, research points us in this direction.

In chapter one, I explain about thoughts, mind, conscious and unconscious mind, and emotions from a neuroscience standpoint. It is my hope that, after you first understand this essential terminology, you will be better able to understand the later chapters.

I then explain how to have a healthy brain and mind. If your brain is not healthy, it cannot function properly. Even if you have the best intention to use your brain, if it is unhealthy, you can't use it in the best way. An unhealthy brain will affect every part of your life.

I describe how the brain affects the body through the nervous, endocrine, and immune systems. I want to clarify for the reader that when I talk in Chapters 3, 4, and 5 about how positive and peaceful thoughts affect our happiness, health, and healing, and how it occurs through the physical and chemical mechanisms in your body. I talk about the science of the brain, mind, thoughts, and emotions and their connection with the body.

My hope is that this book will be informative, inspiring, and practical. The book is organized in the following way. It starts with my story, and then Chapter 1 presents information about the brain and provides some definitions from a neuroscience standpoint. In Chapter 2, I talk about the importance of maintaining a healthy brain and offer suggestions on how to keep the brain healthy in order for it to function better. In Chapter 3, I explain how your thoughts affect your body. Chapter 4 is about positive thoughts, happiness, and optimism. I also talk about depression and its effect on health and healing. In Chapter 5, I talk about the peaceful mind versus the stress response. In Chapter 6, I discuss how your behavior affects your thoughts. Chapter 7 is a summary of the important steps necessary to have a happy, healthy life and what we can all do to heal.

After reading this book, you will:

- Be able to improve your brain's health and function,
- Learn how your thoughts affect your health and healing,
- Be happier and calmer,
- Be healthier and heal faster from any illness,
- Understand that you have control over your happiness, health, and healing, and
- Understand the importance of having a healthy lifestyle; you will consider necessary prevention and medical surgical treatment, but you will not be solely dependent on medication and surgery.

If you control your mind, you can control your body.

How to Use This Book

First of all stay open minded. When I talk about mind and thoughts, I explain them based on neuroscience and biology of the brain. You may have a different opinion and that is ok. My goal is not to approve or disapprove other opinions. My main goal is to show how your thoughts affect your body and how to use them to help to heal yourself.

Reading the whole book gives a sense understanding and confidence on how your brain and thoughts work and how they affect your happiness, health and healing.

Another option is, you can refer to any chapter or section and learn about the specific topic you are interested in. For example, if you are interested in knowing about a peaceful mind and stress, you can read chapter 5. The way I wrote this book, each chapter has its own information, suggestions, and understanding. Each individual chapter does not dependent on reading and understanding other chapters.

My goal is to give you inspiration, motivation and realization that you are the master of your thoughts and therefore your life. You become what you are thinking all day long. Your thoughts manifest in any part of your life. In this book, I especially address the effect of your thoughts on your emotional and physical health.

I also suggest reading this book several times. The more you read the content of this book, the better understanding and clarity you have of what you are looking for.

The more I study neuroscience and how our brain and mind works, the more I appreciate what James Allen wrote in his little master piece *As a Man Thinketh* more than a century ago. I believe his book is must read for everybody.

My goal of this book is nicely summarized by James Allen in the foreword of his book, *As a Man Thinketh*, in 1902,

> *"Its object being to stimulate men and women to*
> *the discovery and perception of the truth,*
> **They themselves are makers of themselves.**
> *By virtue of the thoughts which they choose and encourage;*
> *that the mind is the master weaver, both the inner garment*

of character and the outer garment of circumstances, and that, as they may have hitherto woven in ignorance and pain they may now weave in enlightenment and happiness."

James Allen, 1902

Preface
The Brain Surgeon Who
Had Brain Surgery

I was the third child in a family with six children. My father was a farmer and my mother a housewife. I attended a small village school. I was always very hardworking and focused. I had big dreams. I was so much focused on my studies that I did not know how the years passed. At night I would beg my father to stay up with me a little longer so I wouldn't fall asleep and I would be able to study a little more.

In the morning, when I wanted to get ready for the school, I was reading with my book in my hands while my mother was putting my socks on. The place that my family lived was very warm. I would take my books and go sit under the bridge where it was cool enough to concentrate. Some of the days, I would study for 10 -12 hours. I was the top student during my middle and high school years.

From the beginning, I knew I wanted to help people around me to be happy and healthy. At age five, I decided to become a doctor. I wanted to study abroad. I was always dreaming and thinking about these goals. In my tiny room, I pulled pictures from magazines that kept my dream alive. I would visualize Harvard University, the John Hopkins hospital, the Noble prize.

Living in a tiny Iranian backwater, my father working his way up from a using a donkey, to a motorbike, to a car, I didn't have a clue how these dreams could ever become reality. But they were so real to me that I knew I would get there.

Iranian higher education is government funded for those who qualify academically, so I was able to pass my exams and begin medical school after graduating from high school. I then graduated as the top student from medical school and started general surgery residency in Tehran. I trained in general surgery for one year. Tehran was a thirteen-hour drive from home and I had no family in town. To get by, I literally lived in the call room of the hospital.

Because I graduated the top student from medical school, I was awarded a scholarship to study abroad. I was accepted to study in Toronto, Canada. I cannot describe to you how happy I was. This was my dream! I was in heaven. But there were obstacles to getting a student visa to travel to Canada. For one, I was supposed to be married! But my reputation for focused effort had preceded me and the requirement was officially waved. I was on my way.

Every time I remember my arrival in Toronto, I still feel the wonder and excitement. I had never been outside of Iran. I had never traveled on an airplane. I arrived in Toronto January 5th 1993. It felt like I had arrived on a different planet. There was snow everywhere and holiday decorations on all the shop fronts.

I did not know anybody in Canada. I had to pass an English exam and another medical exam before I was able to begin my residency in neurosurgery.

Diagnosed with a Brain Tumor

I was in my first year of neurosurgery residency in the University of Toronto, Canada. It was December of

1996 and about two weeks before Christmas. One day, my close friend who was one of the senior residents said, "Mahmoud, I don't think you're hearing well in your left ear." I became more concerned when, a few days later, while swimming, I thought water was coming from my left ear. So, I went and saw the ear, nose and throat specialist. He examined me and performed a hearing test. He then ordered an MRI of my brain. As soon as I finished my MRI and came out of the room, the technician who knew me said, "Dr. Rashidi, there is something in your brain's MRI." In fact, I had a large brain tumor called an "acoustic neuroma" that had affected my hearing nerve.

It was a shock. I had a brain tumor. I was alone in Canada. My family was a half a globe away.

After the diagnosis, I talked to one of the surgeons and decided to proceed with surgery. I wanted to be done before Christmas so I could use the holidays for my recovery time and then return to my rotations. I found myself in the same operating room that I had been operating in the day before. Now I was on the operating table. I was feeling humble, scared, and the same time, hopeful. "I have to be strong,"

I told myself. "My mother is waiting to see me back home. I worked so hard and dreamed so many years to get here." Then the anesthesia kicked in and I was out. I woke up in the intensive care unit. I was told my surgery took about 18 hours and everything went well. But the day after surgery, my mouth and throat began to swell and I had difficulty breathing. My doctors tried to put the breathing tube back in, but the swelling was too extreme and they were unable to get it in. They rushed me back to the operating room to do a tracheostomy—to create an opening through the front of my neck directly into the trachea.

The attending surgeon in the operating room was again having difficulty in opening the airway. My blood oxygenation was dropping. Everybody was very tense and unsure about the outcome. Not knowing if I was going to have severe brain damage, or even survive, they tried to reach my family in Iran. Thank God, they were not able to reach my family, because I do not how my family could have stood such news. And what if they had been convinced by the doctors to agree to stop resuscitation? I would be dead now.

Eventually, my friend, a fellow resident who was assisting at the surgery, was able to place the tracheostomy. He also put a chest tube (a flexible tube placed into the chest to drain air) because they thought I may have pneumothorax. He saved my life.

After that, I was in the intensive care unit for days. I was not able to talk. I had to write or point to what I needed. I could feel how completely my life was dependent on the doctors and nurses. The only thing that I had control of was my mind and my thoughts. This was to be a very important realization for me.

I can remember the nurse saying, "Hey, Dr. Rashidi. Can you hear me? Hang in there. You will recover." Those encouraging words were so important for me. I still remember those words. Since then, I always encourage others to hang on and never, ever quit.

I had other complications. I had left facial weakness and I was not to able to close my left eye. I also had a spinal fluid leak from the left side of my nose. But I began to improve. After 2 weeks in the hospital, I rode my bicycle home in the January cold, and came back the next day to continue my residency training. The chairman and head of the department questioned if I would be able to continue my neurosurgery training.

Would I be more comfortable in an easier and shorter residency like emergency medicine? But that was not an option for me. I had been dreaming and working for this since childhood. How could I change my dream now? I *must* heal. I *must* succeed. I was so focused on my goals that I really didn't pay any attention to all those obstacles. Granted, neurosurgery residency is tough. We would start our rounds at 5 am. I would ride my bicycle from home to the hospital. I would change my own dressings (bandages) in front of a mirror by myself.

I was not able to close my left eye due to my left facial palsy. I was using tape to keep my eye closed. But I ended up getting a corneal ulcer, which needed treatment with antibiotics and patching.

I was working with physical therapy for my left facial weakness. I regret I did not work enough with physical therapy. I still have residual weakness on the left side of my face that I am working on. I am sure it will improve.

A few weeks after my surgery I was on call in the hospital and started having a headache. As I mentioned, I had had a small amount of spinal fluid leak from my left nostril after surgery. "I wonder if I could have meningitis due to spinal fluid leak?" I asked myself. By the time I reached the emergency room, **I became unconscious**. One of the neurosurgery residents did a spinal tap. I had bacterial meningitis. I was treated with IV antibiotics. After I recovered from meningitis, I had another surgery to fix the spinal fluid leak.

I Graduated and Began My Practice

I did finish my training successfully and became a fellow of the Royal College of Surgeons of Canada. (FRCSC) I also did a fellowship in pediatric neurosurgery. I completed my training in June 2002.

I moved to the United States and have been practicing in academic and private neurosurgery for sixteen years. I have treated thousands of pediatric and adult patients. I couldn't help notice how a patient's attitude helps their healing. I have many stories of brave patients that kept being positive and how much that affected their healing.

Chapter One
The Human Brain and Mind

"The human brain, then, is the most complicated

organization of matter that we know."

—Isaac Asimov

You, the reader, own the most complex object in the universe, the human brain. Your brain is the center of your thoughts and all higher functions such as imagination, memory, and creativity. It is the home for your consciousness, and the mind forms in your brain.

The human brain weighs about fourteen hundred grams and has a soft tissue consistency like tofu. It is very soft and delicate. I observed how small traction or pressure on the brain caused neurological deficits for the patients after surgery. The brain is located in the cranium (the top portion of the skull), and it is protected more than any other organ in the body. The brain floats in cerebrospinal

1

fluid. Our brain receives information from the outside world through our sensory organs.

The brain contains a hundred billions neurons with trillions of connections which, through a complex electrical and chemical activity, allows us to think, feel and experience the world. All life experiences and memories are stored in the brain.

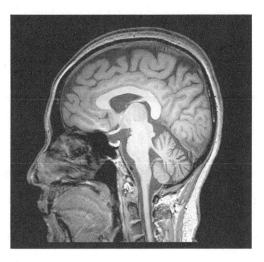

Your brain is the center of everything you do such as breathing, storing all your memories, talking and walking, feelings, learning any skills and making any decision. **Simply, your brain makes you, you.**

Damage to the brain can affect a part of or an entire person's life. I have seen many patients with trauma or stroke in the frontal lobe where their whole personality has changed. They literally can become a different person with a different personality. Their family sometimes blames the patient and asks why they are behaving so differently, but it's the patient's brain that does that.

These changes could be temporary until the brain returns to normal or, it could be permanent if damage is severe and the structure of the brain has changed. I remember a patient who was an accountant. When she had a fall and developed a blood clot over her brain, she was not able to calculate simple addition or subtraction, things that an elementary student can do. If our brains do not function properly, it can affect every part of our life from simple actions like talking and moving, to higher functions, such as thinking and decision making.

Your brain wants to learn anything you experience, such as reading, hearing, seeing and doing. Your brain is essential for everything you learn. Your networks of neurons, unlike the computer electrical connections, are flexible and you can change the network. When you learn, your brain learns. Your brain learns with change in chemical and electrical activity in its huge network. When you become a master at any skill, the structure of the brain permanently changes and you will not be able to unlearn it easily or at all.

That's the reason why it is so difficult to change. When you want to change, your brain structure has to change; otherwise the change is temporary as long as it is in the working memory. This is the reason that a lot of people promise to do or not to do something and then they act just like before; because their brain has not changed yet, and blaming them would not be helpful. They need to persist and act the way they want to be and, over time, their brain will rewire and become a new brain, and as the result, they become a new person.

Thoughts

Thinking is an essential function of the human brain. Each animal has an essential function that helps it survive and become proficient at what it does. For humans, our special function is thinking.

What are thoughts? The act of thinking about something that produces an idea or opinion is called a thought. When we have a thought, electrical signals travel back and forth between the neurons related to that thought. Every time these neurons communicate with each other, it becomes easier for them to communicate in the future.

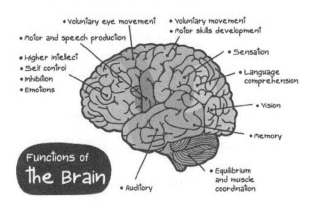

What thought is going to be in your brain at each moment? It depends on your attention. Your mind flits from one thought to another. This thought could be related to internal or external stimuli. For example, when you look at a picture, you have thoughts related to that picture. If you hear a noise, your brain will start thinking about that noise. You can also think about an idea in the past or the future. It seems as sensations and ideas are constantly fighting to get your attention. Your thought at each moment therefore depends on the dominant neuronal network in your brain that you pay attention to.

To make my point clear, I am going to do a short test to see whether I can get your attention and therefore control the kind of thought in your mind over the next few seconds as you read the next few sentences. Think about each question for a few seconds before going to the next.

- What is the color of your front door?
- What did you do last New Year's Eve?
- What are you going to do tomorrow?

During the time you were reading the above questions, your stream of thoughts went from present to past and then to future.

The neuronal activations in the brain fluctuate as waves. These electrical activities can be displayed in brain waves in EEG (electroencephalogram). Brain waves are measured in cycles per second or Hertz. These waves from high to low speed are as follows;

- Gamma waves: gamma waves are the fastest brain waves. They are as the result of simultaneous information processing from different parts of the brain. They have the subtlest frequency and pass the information rapidly and quietly. These waves exist continually in the brain in all mental states, except during deep, non-dreaming sleep.

- Beta waves: beta waves are dominant during waking hours of our life when we are having a cognitive task. For example, when we think intensively, as in, having a serious conversation or giving a speech.

- Alpha waves: alpha waves are slower than beta waves and are dominant when the brain is at rest and calm and at present moment. Examples are some meditative states and activities like gardening when thoughts quietly flow.

- Theta waves: the next slower-frequency brain waves are called theta waves. Theta waves occur during sleep, deep meditation and daydreaming.

- Delta waves: the slowest brain waves are delta waves. They occur during deep, dreamless sleep. In this state there is no external awareness.

These brain waves will never go down to zero, because that would mean the brain is dead. This would result in a flat EEG, which shows the absence of brain waves.

Why information about brain waves is important? As you noticed above, the brain has different brain waves in different external and internal states. Balance in brain waves is important for emotional health and behavior. Over arousal in certain parts of the brain can cause anxiety and under arousal can lead to depression.

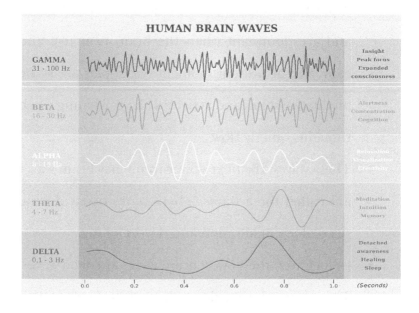

The dominant thoughts that flow in your mind depend on your experiences and your attention. Most of the time, due to your habits, you pay attention to familiar situations. You have thousands of thoughts a day which are called stream or train of thoughts. These thoughts are mostly similar thoughts to ones you had the day before, because most of your thoughts are also habitual. You pay attention by habit and do the same things over and over.

> *"All thinking is based, in part, on prior convictions."*
> —George A. Kelly

The good news is that you don't have to be a creature of your habits.

You can change and choose different thoughts. You are the master. You can control your mind, and it is up to you to either use this amazing power or let your mind control you. With this power, you have control over your happiness, peace, health, healing, relationship, and finances.

The Mind

What is the mind? There is no single, agreed upon definition of the mind. From a neuroscience and biology standpoint; the mind is the flow of thought that is the result of electrical and chemical activities of the neurons and between them in the brain.

The mind is a result of the function of the brain. Therefore the mind is a state that occurs when the brain is alive and at work. An injury to the brain affects the mind. When the brain is not alive and is not working, there is no mind.

In this book, when I talk about the brain, I refer more to the physical brain in the cranium, but when I talk about the mind, I refer to the functional aspect of the brain.

When does your mind control you? When you let the beliefs and thoughts in your mind determine your behavior, your feeling and emotions without effort to change them.

How do you control your mind? You basically control your thoughts. You do not have to think about something that you do not want to think. You start thinking about something else. You can get some help from outside like music, a picture, talking to somebody, making a phone call, anything that changes the state of your mind.

What does it mean to change the state of your mind? It simply means you change your thought by thinking about something else. You use a different neuronal network in your brain. You can choose which neuronal network to use and you can do it with attention to things you want. The more you use a neuronal network, the easier it becomes to use it next time. Sometimes, after mostly thinking about the things you want, it becomes easier to bounce back to positive if your thoughts become negative.

Consciousness and Unconsciousness

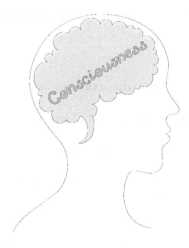

Consciousness

Consciousness implies awareness of experiences of the external and internal world. Consciousness is essential to understanding and making decisions regarding your free will and your choices. Your view of reality, of the universe, and of yourself depends on consciousness. The conscious mind is the thinking mind.

Consciousness has different levels.

A person in coma or deep sleep has no consciousness, then to drowsiness, that has some consciousness to alert that he/she is conscious.

What are the content of our consciousness at any moment?

At each moment, the content of our consciousness depends on our perception. Our perception depends on our expectation and sensory information that our brain receives. Our expectations affect our conscious awareness. For example, when you are looking around, you are not conscious to everything in your visual field. It depends on your visual expectation. You only see what your brain expects or wants to see. It is the best guess of reality.

What is self-consciousness?

Self-consciousness is the awareness of oneself. It has several components; for example:

- Bodily self-conscious; that means we are aware of our body.
- Narrative self-conscious; that I am aware of my past, present and future.
- Social self-conscious; I am aware of me and others are separate from me.

We are conscious because of the complex electrical activities among the neurons. Consciousness is not related to one part of the brain; it is the coordinated activity of many parts of the brain.

Because consciousness comes from the complex activities of neurons, the process of consciousness is slower than the process of unconsciousness. How the biological machine inside our head gives us the consciousness is not well known.

Unconsciousness

Unconsciousness is a much larger part of the mind. About 80 to 90 percent of the mind is unconsciousness.

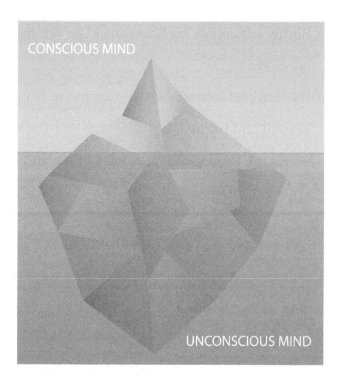

Unconscious mind is beyond our awareness. Most of our mental life is unconscious. The heartbeat and breathing and other automated activities in the body are unconscious. All habitual activities are unconscious and most of our activities during our lives are habitual.

The unconscious is the storehouse for all your memories and experiences. These memories and experiences make you who you are. These memories and experiences form the beliefs and habits that run your life. When we do something habitually and unconsciously, the brain does not use that much energy and effort. It is a short cut neuronal circuit. The habit has already been programed in the brain. This is the reason it is much easier to act habitually; unless we pay attention and be conscious to what we are doing, otherwise we will continue to act based on our habits, just like we have done before.

There is no chance to change, unless, consciously, we choose different behaviors and become committed to act on the new behavior for about 60 days without interruption.

Every new activity that we learn initially is conscious, but after being learned, it will go into long-term memory and the unconscious. This process frees you up to be able to pay attention to the next things you need to learn.

For example, when you first wanted to drive, initially, it seemed difficult to think about how to do many things at the same time; use the brakes, look around, and turn.

The reason it was so difficult is that you had to do all these activities consciously.

But after some time spent driving, most people not only drive, but also talk, eat, drink, and put on their makeup (bad idea) without any problem. At this stage, most of these activities are done unconsciously. This process is necessary for the brain so it will be more efficient. That's why routine activities are stored in the unconscious part of our minds, leaving our consciousness and thoughts free to learn new skills.

The Emotions and Feelings

In this section, you will find out where is the center of emotions and feelings in the brain.

Is there any difference between emotion and feeling?

The emotions such as fear and anger reflect and interplay between cortical areas, such as prefrontal cortex, cingulate gyrus, and subcortical regions, such as the hypothalamus and amygdala. The stimuli may integrate by subcortical structure like amygdala, and trigger immediate autonomic and endocrine responses. These responses are such as facial expressions and muscle contractions, and prepare us for a physical response.

These immediate responses are at an unconscious level. When the cerebral cortex becomes involved, it results in a conscious experience of emotion, and that is feeling. The cortex also sends the signal to the subcortical area and enhances or suppresses the somatic manifestations of emotions. This is a level of conscious control and we regulate our response to the stimuli, therefore we can control our responses to what bothers us. This is important in stress management and avoids violent behavior when, for example, we are angry.

Most scientists believe the primary emotions are fear, anger, sadness, and joy. Neuroscientist, Antonio Damasio, adds surprise and disgust to the primary emotions.

The other emotions are secondary; these are learned emotions, like guilt or shame.

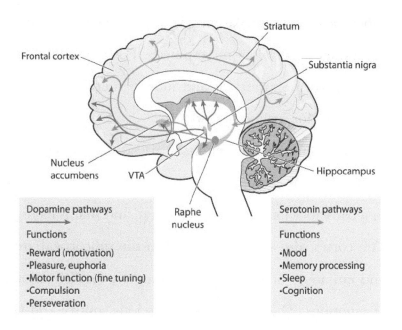

Feelings

Feelings are private and inward; they register at a mostly conscious level. Feelings help you deal with the problem that is signaled by emotions. It means you feel the emotion. When a stimulus produces an emotion by activating amygdala, for example, fear, then when the cortex becomes activated, we feel the fear.

Chapter Two
Healthy Brain and Mind

"There is no health without mental health."

—David Satcher

The Importance of Brain Health

The brain controls every moment of your life (of course, mostly unconsciously). Beyond automatic (unconscious) activities, all your conscious work comes from the brain. All higher functions like thinking, decision-making, memory, and creativity happen in the brain. Therefore, for having a productive life we need a healthy brain.

The brain is the most special organ in the body. Life continues as long as the brain is healthy and functioning. Death happens after the brain stops functioning. The lungs or heart may stop, but the patient dies because oxygen and glucose do not get to the brain.

We have an amazing brain, but at same time it is fragile and we need to take care of it. The health of the brain affects its performance and as the result, our performance in all areas of our life. It will affect our learning, our job, decision-making, and our relationships. The health of the brain is very important at any age. It even becomes more crucial and obvious at old age. I have seen many patients who suffer from the diseases and conditions that have affected their brain from depression, substance abuse, to dementia associated with Alzheimer's disease, stroke and head injury.

I have seen the significant loss as the result of brain damage. I have seen many patients with dementia who were very smart and highly accomplished people when they were younger. They were engineers, businessmen, teachers and many other jobs. They had successful lives, but now, with dementia, they may not remember the name of their grandchildren or even recognize them.

Many families who look after their elderly members with dementia realize how important the health of the brain is. These younger members of the family can learn not only to take care of their own brain, but also help the family members with dementia. Dementia progresses over time, and there are some factors that make it progress faster or slower. We can help our elderly family members to keep their brain healthier and more functional. For all these reasons, I dedicate this whole chapter for how to keep our brain healthy.

Basic Anatomy of a Human Brain

Knowing some basic structure of your brain helps you to understand your brain and its functions better. You will also have a better understanding of how to take care of your brain's health. Once you have some information about the brain, you are not following my suggestions blindly, and you will be more informed and motivated. I believe everybody needs to know the basic structure and function of the human brain. It's worth your time and effort and it will pay in a big way in the future. I made it easy for you to understand it and not get too bored. Here you are, enjoy some anatomy of your amazing brain.

The brain can be divided into three parts. Each part has a different function.

1. **Hindbrain,** which is located in the base of the skull and is the first part of the brain that has evolved. The hindbrain has three structures; the medulla oblongata, pons, and cerebellum.

   Medulla Oblongata: The automatic behaviors that keep us alive, such as breathing and heart beat are located in medulla oblongata.

   Pons also controls vital functions such as heart beat, breathing and sleep.

   The cerebellum, or small brain, is involved in the sense of the body's position and movement. It is also linked to emotion and cognition.

2. **Midbrain**, many physical actions such as hearing and eye movements happen in the midbrain.

3. **Forebrain** which includes the cerebral cortex, thalamus, hypothalamus, hippocampus, amygdala, basal ganglia.

   - Cerebral cortex is the outer layer that envelopes cerebral hemispheres. It is folded inside the skull. If it spread flat, it covers 1.6 square meters. Human cerebral cortex is much larger than in any other animal. It is thought that the cerebral cortex makes us human. The human cerebral cortex is the center for higher functions, including reason, language, and conscious thinking. All our decisions are made in the cortex of the brain.

The cerebrum has two hemispheres, right and left, also known as right and left brain. Each hemisphere has four principle lobes. The **frontal lobes** are the place for individual personalities, thinking and planning. The **parietal lobes** are responsible for sensory integration. The **temporal lobes** are involved with auditory information and language. The **occipital lobes** are the place for visual cortex.

The two halves of the brain are connected to each other with the corpus callosum, the largest nerve bundle in the brain, made up of about two hundred million neurons (nerve cells).

In some of the cases, for controlling seizure, the surgeon cuts the corpus callosum (called corpus colostomy) for limiting the spread of epileptic activity between the two halves of the brain. In some cases, with cutting the connection of the two halves of the brain, caused the split of the unity of brain function, and then as the body is controlled by two independent brains. For example, a smoker reported, after this surgery, he was experiencing different functioning with his right and left hands. When he reached a cigarette with his right hand, his left hand would grab the cigarette and throw it away.

- Thalamus is a relay station and directs the sensory information to the cortex.
- Hypothalamus is responsible for the control and integration of endocrine function, thermoregulation, also has role in behavior and memory.
- Hippocampus is important for long-term memory.
- Amygdala is the emotional center.
- Basal ganglia are important in motor behavior and learning.

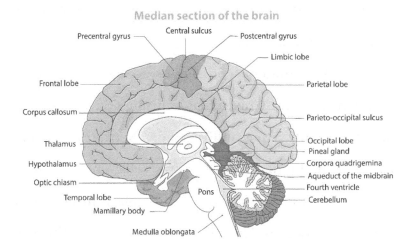

The brain has two types of cells: neurons or nerve cells, and neuroglia, or supporting cells. The neuron has three parts:

1. **Cell body**,
2. **Dendrites;** an array of branching fibers that extend from cell body,
3. **Axon;** another fiber that extends from the end of the cell body.

The electrical signals flow in one direction. The information gathers by dendrites and transfers through axon to other neurons. Neurons communicate through a tiny gap, called a synapse. They use chemical messengers called neurotransmitters.

Neurotransmitters send signals across the synapses between neurons. This signal transmission is very fast and takes only a few milliseconds. Neurotransmitters excite or inhibit the receiving nerve cells. Therefore, the transmissions between neurons take place in electrical and chemical stages. These flows of information ultimately make up our thoughts and feelings.

Dozens of neurotransmitters have been identified, including serotonin, dopamine, and norepinephrine. Different transmitters have different actions and certain transmitters are related to mental and physical health. Disorders of some transmitters are linked to emotional and neurological illnesses.

For example, the neurotransmitter, dopamine, is essential for movement control. A deficiency in dopamine is associated with slowness of movement and other symptoms of Parkinson's disease. Dopamine is also the transmitter for reward- motivated behavior and it is necessary for learning and addiction. The neurotransmitter, Serotonin, is linked to depression and anxiety.

Brain Plasticity

We know now that the brain is soft-wired throughout our life, not hard-wired, as once thought. We need a healthy brain for proper brain maturation. For example, for forming new brain cells and new connections, we need certain nutrients. For making the transmitters, we need protein and essential fatty acids.

Foods that contain anti-oxidants, such as berries, are very important, especially in older age; they keep the brain faculties active. Physical activities are very important for brain plasticity at any age. Let's learn more about brain plasticity which is very important in context of learning new skills and change.

I want to show you how you can restructure your brain the way you want. You do not have to be stuck with the way your brain structured during your childhood by somebody else. Do not wait another minute, start changing the thoughts, beliefs, and habits which you do

not want with changing the structure of your brain. I will show you how to do it in some practical ways.

Brain plasticity means that neuronal interactions are capable of rewiring. The brain can make new connections, and new brain cells can recover. Although brain plasticity is the most obvious during childhood, the brain remains malleable through your lifetime. With learning and experience, your brain has the capacity to change its structure and its function.

Brain plasticity gives you the ability to learn and memorize information. During a lifetime of educational experiences, brain cells make new connections, and the new connections mean learning. Each neuron can make a connection with up to thousands of other neurons (nerve cells). The brain has about a hundred billion neurons and can have up to a hundred trillion connections.

The Brain Increases Connections as You Learn

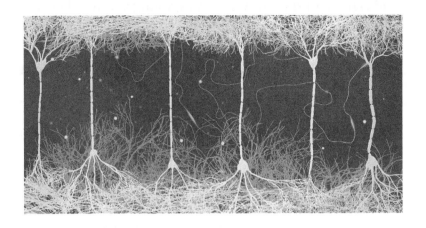

Brain plasticity begins during development and continues throughout a lifetime. Neuronal connections gradually mature during childhood and peak in early adolescence. Sensory and motor skills mature first; judgment and impulse control mature in the prefrontal cortex later.

This is why adolescents often have difficulty with impulse control and make decisions from the emotional part of the brain; there is a lag between the emotional and cognitive area of the brain maturation.

For wise judgment, there is a need for balance between different regions of the brain. Until the age of five to six years old, there is not a good connection between the left and right hemisphere. Sometimes, young children become confused because they cannot connect the information received by the right brain with the information received by the left brain.

One of the amazing things is that our experiences and learning affect the brain's plasticity. Therefore, we can have self-directed plasticity. By learning and thinking in a special program or experiment, the related neuronal network makes more connections and the area of the brain related to that work may grow larger. For example, analyzing of Einstein's brain revealed some distinctive physical characteristics. The area of his brain related to mathematical abilities and special reasoning was significantly larger. The neurons may have been more closely connected, which would allow them to work more effectively.

The plasticity of the brain is also very important for recovery after damage to the brain, such as a head injury or a stroke. As a neurosurgeon, I've seen patients with severe head injuries who were comatose and in intensive care for weeks or months. But the same person, one year later, would walk into my office. The reason is the brain's plasticity.

Brain plasticity can cause the recovery of behavior that was lost because of the head injury or stroke. Because of plasticity, some brain cells can recover, and some neurons make new connections. Also, some of the neurons can become active and take over the functions of the lost neurons.

In some cases, patients have weakness or a problem with speech after a stroke. These same patients, after weeks or months, may recover completely. This is due to the brain's plasticity.

I would like to mention here the importance of rehabilitation. The most important factor for using the power of our brain plasticity is practice. Rehabilitation is crucial for patients with a head injury. Brain plasticity and neuron recovery takes time. It is important that the patient continues proper rehabilitation until the nerve cells recover. Patients should imagine that they have recovered. For example, my patients that have weakness of the arm or leg after a head injury or stroke, when they are lying down in the bed and I tell them, "imagine that your weakness has improved and you are using the arm or leg." This imagination activates the neurons related to that motion and helps them heal faster.

The Aging Brain

The brain ages gradually, and this aging process is associated with some structural, chemical and functional changes in the brain. If the brain matures healthy with wisdom that comes from experience, the elderly brain has better judgment. In a healthy elderly brain, except the bit of reduction in the speed of processing information, most other higher functions of the brain stay stable.

With age, some of the neurons die and also, there is a decrease in some of the transmitters. But if the brain stays healthy and active in old age, because of neuroplasticity, the most active and useful neurons and connections remain intact. With new learning, more new connections will be made. Therefore, mental activities are very important for keeping the brain healthy and functional.

Only a small percentage of the population will be affected by dementia, including Alzheimer's disease, which we do not know the exact cause or prevention of. Most other dementias are due to some preventable factors, such as depression, diet, sleep, and medication side effects.

The good news is that with our behavior, we can delay the effects and severity of the progression of aging and cognitive decline. We can have a healthier brain and mind at any age.

How to Keep the Brain Healthy

The brain is about 2 percent of the total body weight, but it consumes 20 percent of the body's oxygen and glucose at any moment. The brain is dependent on a constant supply of oxygen and glucose. Most of this energy is keeping the brain ready for action by maintaining the electrical field in the brain.

When a person's blood pressure drops, for example, on a hot summer day, the brain does not receive enough glucose and oxygen temporarily and he/she may become dizzy or faint. Because the neurons cannot produce enough electrical activities, the person loses consciousness and falls on the ground. Then, enough blood goes to the brain and he/she regains consciousness. If the brain does not receive oxygen and glucose for more than three to five minutes, brain cells may die and cause a stroke.

The brain's prime function is keeping the body safe and ready for action at any moment. The brain, as a source of mental function, works better in a healthy body; therefore, a healthy heart is linked to a healthy brain. Whatever you do to keep your heart healthy will also keep your brain healthy.

The important factors for a healthy brain include nutrition, physical activity, sleep, social activities, and brain and mind stimulation.

Nutrition

The type of the food that our ancestors were eating was important in the human brain growth. When the tools were developed to kill animals around 2 million years ago, it was essential in the expansion of the human brain. Meat is a rich source of nutrients. Also, fire was important for the growth of the human brain, since it allow us to get more nutrients from our food.

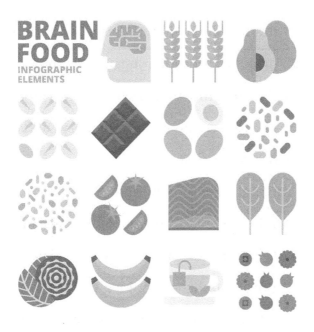

The type of food you consume shapes your body and behavior. The structure and function of your brain is affected by your diet.

A good diet is important for a healthy brain. A healthy diet is as important for brain health as it is for the heart and the rest of the body. A healthy and balanced diet will help maintain brain chemistry at the healthy level that is necessary for optimal brain function.

Here are some important factors that are necessary for optimal brain health and function:

1. Hydration; about 80 percent of the brain is water, so lack of hydration negatively impacts brain health and function. Dehydration causes mood disturbance, can impair memory, and reduces cognitive function.

2. Antioxidants are important for brain health and can be found in vegetables (especially green, leafy vegetables) and fruits (especially berries). Antioxidants help cognitive functions. They get rid of toxins known as free radicals. A free radical is any atom or molecule with a single, unpaired electron that seeks to pair with another electron from another molecule. This makes the other molecule unstable. It starts a chain of reactions that may cause damage to DNA, protein, or cells. In this way, antioxidants protect the brain cells from an early death. Blueberries and strawberries contain flavonoids which delay the cognitive decline.

3. Omega 3 is an essential fatty acid. Omega 3 can improve mood and help cognitive function.

   The following foods have high level of omega 3:

Salmon	Caviar
Sardines	Walnuts
Herring	Flaxseeds
Mackerel	Chia seeds
Oysters	Soybeans

4. Docosahexaenoic acid (DHA) is an omega 3 fatty acid. Our body needs DHA for a healthy brain. DHA is important for the myelin sheath. Myelin sheath is a wrapping fatty tissue that covers a neuron's axon. It insulates and protects the axon and increases the speed of impulse transmissions. DHA can prevent cognitive decline in patients with Alzheimer's disease. Foods with a high level of DHA also have high levels of omega 3, like salmon, halibut, sardines, tuna, herring, oysters, and trout.

5. Proteins and amino acids: Proteins provide the brain with amino acids, which are necessary for

synthesizing neurotransmitters. Good proteins help to boost the level of neurotransmitters like serotonin and dopamine, which help you feel happy and reduce depression and anxiety. **Choline**, an amino acid found in egg yolk, is necessary for manufacturing the neurotransmitter acetylcholine, which is important for your memory.

Sources of protein:

- Fish and shellfish
- Dairy products like cottage cheese, yogurt, and milk
- Beef and lamb
- Eggs
- Tofu and soy products
- Nuts and seeds
- Peanut butter
- Beans

6. Vitamins D and E: Vitamin E is a very important antioxidant; it neutralizes free radicals. It is especially good for older patients and patients with dementia.

Some good sources of vitamin E:

- Walnuts

- Almonds

- Sunflower seeds

- Whole wheat

- Sweet potatoes

A List of Healthy Foods for the Brain

Leafy Greens	Vegetables	Fruits
▪ spinach	▪ broccoli	▪ berries
▪ collard greens	▪ pumpkin	▪ cherries
▪ kale	▪ bell peppers	▪ apple
▪ romaine	▪ asparagus	▪ grapes
▪ Swiss chard	▪ red onion	▪ lemon
Proteins	**Oils**	**Seeds and Nuts**
▪ egg	▪ olive oil	▪ almonds
▪ salmon	▪ canola oil	▪ walnuts
▪ trout	▪ sunflower oil	▪ sunflower seeds
▪ shrimp	▪ coconut oil	▪ cocoa powder
▪ mackerel	▪ soybean oil	▪ peanuts

Try Not to Harm Your Brain

- Limit sugar. The brain needs glucose, and there is

  nothing to be concerned about with a small amount

  of sugar, but too much of this energy source can

be bad for the brain. Most people eat too much sugar. It has been shown that there is a link between excess glucose and impaired memory and cognitive function.

- Avoid drugs that damage the brain.

- Avoid marijuana; some studies suggest regular use of marijuana in adolescents causes impairment in memory, learning, and impulse control.

- Avoid opioids like heroin; long-term use of heroin causes changes in the prefrontal cortex and medial temporal lobe. These changes are associated with impaired memory and behavior control.

- Stimulants like cocaine cause damage to the brain.

- Alcohol; prolonged alcohol abuse can cause brain damage.

- Smoking reduces oxygen supply to the brain. Smoking can promote neurodegenerative illnesses, like Alzheimer's disease.

- Avoid activities that have a high risk of head injury.

- Drive carefully, and use a helmet when riding a motorcycle or bicycle. I have seen many adolescent and young patients with head injuries; their lives were changed forever.

Physical Activity

Exercise can change the brain and enhance brain power. Exercise increases the level of growth factor in the brain and helps make new neurons and new connections. Exercise also increases oxygenation to the brain. Physical activity increases production of neurotransmitters like serotonin, dopamine, and norepinephrine. They help to improve mood and happiness.

Exercise increases the level of the neurotransmitters GABA and serotonin. These specific neurotransmitters help improve anxiety and depression. When you exercise, it is like taking antidepressant medication, which increases the serotonin level in your brain.

Physical activity plays a role in the prevention and treatment of depression. For example, if you are depressed and feel like staying on the sofa, the best thing you could do is go for a walk; it will improve the left prefrontal cortex activity, and you will feel more joy.

Physical activity is beneficial for mood, memory, and learning. Exercise helps neurogenesis (development and growth of new neurons) in the hippocampus, which is important for long-term memory.

In school, physical activity helps children to learn and memorize better. If you are trying to learn new material, a short exercise can give you immediate benefit. For example, taking a 10 minute exercise will help you memorize easier a list of 30 nouns compared to sitting around. Short, intensive bursts of exercise are very effective when you are learning.

Exercise helps the release of transmitters that are involved in forming new neuronal connections. We learn by making new connections between neurons.

Most physicians recommend thirty minutes of moderate, aerobic physical activity a day, five days a week.

Moderate aerobic exercise includes walking, swimming, even mowing the lawn. The goal is thirty minutes of physical activity every day. Studies of people with long and happy lives showed they had physical activities that they loved and enjoyed, like gardening or walking in nature.

It is very important that the exercise is done with positive feelings.

Whenever you feel down, anxious, or depressed, go for a walk or start a physical activity. It will improve your mood.

Exercise also reduces stress by decreasing cortisol levels, which increase when under stress. In the treatment of PTSD and anxiety, exercise should be part of the treatment protocol. It is important to make regular physical activity part of your daily lifestyle.

Sleep

On average, a person that lives for 75 years spends 1/3 of it, or 25 years, sleeping.

Why do we sleep for several hours a day?

It is mostly a mystery, but it is crucial to our survival. If people do not sleep for a few days, they start hallucinating and may have seizures. There are several theories for why we spend several hours a day sleeping:

1. The brain repairs itself during sleep.

2. During sleep, the waste products are being cleared from the brain.

3. Some of the scientists suggesting, during sleep, the connection (synapses) between neurons slow down and even get smaller, so that the brain does not become overloaded with memories.

It is possible that sleep has several functions.

There is evidence that sleep could be localized in some part of the brain. For example, the most active region of the brain during waking hours could sleep longer and deeper.

Sleep is crucial for maintaining a healthy, functioning brain. If you do not have adequate, regular sleep, it will negatively affect your brain in several ways.

Sleep is necessary for:

- Myelin formation (a myelin sheath covers the axon of the neuron and increases the speed of nerve impulses)
- Certain genetic processes
- Protein synthesis

Lack of sleep affects concentration and the absorption of new information. It has been shown that when schoolchildren are woken up a few times in the night, the day after, they have problems with concentration and are more anxious and reactive.

We Need Sleep for Learning

Dreaming is important for memory and emotional health. When we dream, it seems that the brain talks to itself at a level different from being consciously awake. Dreams often relate to recent experiences during waking hours. Dreaming is important for storing, organizing and consolidating our memories. During a dream, the brain solves emotional conflicts that happened during the waking hours.

People with lack of sleep will be more irritable, more tired and more prone to stress. Even partial deprivation will affect the mood. Our mood influences how much we enjoy our life. When we are in a good mood, we feel that we can do anything, and small, daily setbacks do not get us down. But when we are in a bad mood, we become irritated over small things and can't enjoy our life.

Sleep deprivation affects the brain health and mental ability. When we are sleepy, we make more mistakes. For example, driving when moderately sleep deprived affects the brain function equivalent to driving while drunk. Sleep need varies as we age, and for each individual.

The U.S. National Sleep Foundation recommendations are as follows:

- School age children 6-13 years old: 9-11 hours
- Teenagers 14-17 years old: 8-10 hours
- Adults 18-64 years old: 7-9 hours
- Older adults 65+ years old: 7-8 hours

One hour less or more than above recommendation may be appropriate.

For example, 6-10 for adults may be appropriate.

There are several methods to improve sleep: proper diet, a cool and quiet bedroom, light exposure during the day, and exercise. Exercise not only increases sleep time, it also increases deep sleep.

Social Activities

Socialization is very important for the health of the brain, especially in old age. During a social activity, mirror neurons are activated, and their activity helps cognition (A mirror neuron is a neuron that fires both when we act and when we observe the same action performed by others). In older people, socialization reduces cognitive decline and helps memory.

Isolated humans have a higher risk of dementia. It is important for older people, and even people with dementia, to remain part of their community. They should spend time with their family and friends. Family members are usually busy and scattered. We need to prioritize family time. It does not need to be formal or a big arrangement, we can just get together for tea, play a game, or a chat.

We should try to visit our older parents as frequently as possible, especially if they are in the nursing homes. Take them out for a dinner or the places they have old memories at. It is also important that older people spend time with younger adults and children. It would make them emotionally, intellectually and physiologically younger.

Social activities activate the social part of the brain that includes the olfactory and the cingulate cortexes. When you help others, mirror neurons are activated in your own brain, and you conclude that you can help yourself. That brings a sense of well-being. When you have empathy and compassion for others, you have compassion for yourself.

Thus, insensitivity is bad for your mental health. When we are kind to others, it is not only increasing transmitters in their brain, which elevates their mood, but also, kindness does the same thing in our brain (the person who acts kindly) and the brain of the observer of that act of kindness.

One of my suggestions for people with depression is that when you are feeling down, do not stay alone and feel sorry for yourself. Get out talk to somebody, even better, if you can, help somebody.

Caring for others and being cared for has a positive effect on your brain. In children, lack of nurturing can cause neurochemical abnormalities. For example, babies whose mothers are less attentive, such as the children of mothers with depression, risk having behavioral problems later in life.

The Brain and Mental Stimulation

The brain improves with use. Mental stimulation is necessary for brain health. Brain stimulation changes the brain through plasticity. Brain stimulation starts early, likely in the womb, and causes brain development. If the brain does not receive enough stimulation in the early childhood, some of the functions of the brain may not develop enough later on in life.

The human brain can be stimulated by reading, writing, and learning a new language, as well as creative activities like music and art. We usually like to engage in familiar activities that are passive and mostly related to the subcortical area of the brain. These activities do not help brain development that much. But learning new and complex information will activate the cortex and forming new neuronal connections. Therefore, it promotes the development of a brain reserve. Well-developed brains are more resistant to neurodegenerative disease, like Alzheimer's, later in life.

Lack of mental fitness can reduce mental function, just as the lack of physical exercise causes muscles to atrophy. Enriched environments stimulate the brain's neuronal networks and as a result, a healthier and better functioning brain for a life time.

Having a lifelong learning process will keep your brain sharp. Read or listen to new and different ideas, even it is uncomfortable, it is not only good for brain health, it will also expand your mind.

Adapt a Healthy Brain Life Style

Now that you are familiar with the important factors for having a healthy brain, look at your life and find out which of these factors are missing or are not enough in your life style. You are most likely doing some of these activities in life, so add some other factors and avoid the activities that may damage your brain. Your brain is dynamic; even you have been doing something harmful up until now, and if you stop doing it, your brain will repair itself. It is never too late start doing what is healthier for your brain.

A Healthy Mind

A healthy body requires a healthy mind. The health of the mind and brain are interconnected and affect each other.

A clear mind is a mind without confusion and too many negative thoughts. It is a mind in balance. A clear mind can help you find a way through life and help you see situations with greater clarity. In a clear mind, the stream of thoughts can flow smoothly and in the direction of your goals, without too many interruptions. With a clear mind, you will have better concentration and make better decisions.

How to Keep Your Mind Healthy and Clear

Having an orderly mind without confusion is very important. If there is something of concern happening in your life, you need to be sure to keep it in its own place and not extend it to another part of your life. For example, if you have a problem in your relationship, you need to think about it and spend a certain amount of time on it. If it consumes your mind and thoughts too much, you may ignore your health or your work. You may make other mistakes that cause even more problems and more stress and confusion.

Negative thoughts and feelings clutter the mind. Replace hate with love, anger with gentleness and calmness, and fear with faith. A pure mind and pure thoughts, a beautiful mind, will produce these qualities through your actions.

If you want to have a pure and beautiful life, have a pure and beautiful mind.

Two important factors in having a healthy and clear mind are forgiveness and mindfulness.

Forgiveness

Forgiveness is essential for mental health. Resentment affects the thought process and how you perceive the world. Forgiving yourself and others causes you to release stress and gives you a peaceful mind. A clear and peaceful mind is not possible without forgiveness. With forgiveness, you cut the rope that holds you back, and you make yourself free. Forgiveness reduces anxiety, stress, and depression. It helps improve the immune system and your health.

You can learn to be more forgiving of others. You need to make a conscious decision to let go of negative feelings and resentment, whether the other person deserves it or not. Forgiveness helps others, but it is really for your own health and healing.

There is no limit for how many times you should forgive. Every day is a new day and it should be a new day for the mind too, otherwise, your mental and emotional energy will be used for yesterday. Instead of being present in the moment, doing your best at your present day, you will be stuck in the hurt of yesterday. Learn from the event and let it go, instead of dwelling on how hurtful it was.

Mindfulness

Mindfulness is a mental state of being aware and conscious of the present moment. When you are mindful, you are fully present in the moment and aware of where you are and what you are doing, without being overly reactive or being overwhelmed with the situation around you. Most people's minds are not in the present time. Their minds are filled with worry, fear, anger, and regret. This is forgetfulness, not mindfulness.

Fear and worry about the future, or feeling guilt or shame about the past, affects the clarity of the mind.

In a mindful state, the prefrontal cortex is activated and therefore inhibits the over activity of the amygdala (emotional center) and sympathetic nervous system. Therefore, the mind and the body become calm. In this state, you do not focus on the stressful part of an experience. Mindfulness gives you an open focus and shifts your brain from a narrow focus, which is a characteristic of stress. Mindfulness also includes carefulness and alertness.

How Can You Achieve Mindfulness?

You naturally possess mindfulness, but when you practice it, it becomes more available to you. Whenever you become aware of your experiences with your senses, or become aware of thoughts and feelings, you are mindful. In mindfulness, the mind and body are in sync. You can train your brain to be mindful. With practicing mindfulness, our brain makes new neuronal connections and networks. As a result, we adapt a new way thinking to promote peace of mind.

Mindful practices include:

- Mindful meditation,
- Silence,
- Mindful breathing,
- Becoming aware of your body,
- Mindful walking.

Chapter Three
The Effects of Thoughts
on the Body

"The body is a delicate and plastic instrument, which responds readily to the thoughts by which it is impressed, and the habits of thought will produce their own effects, good or bad, upon it."

—James Allen

Thoughts Affect Health and Healing

The effects of the thoughts on the health and healing have been discussed for a long time. This topic has been described in the religious books and by philosophers and psychologists. In recent years, neuroscientists have discovered much more about the interconnection of the thoughts, the brain and the body. A large number of the emotional and physical diseases are related to our thought life.

Thoughts are real things. Thoughts have a biological basis; basically, the neurons carry electrical activity and communicate with other neurons. When you have a thought, you have electrical and chemical activities in certain networks of your brain. We can detect these electrical activities in different brain imaging.

These activated neurons in turn activate the emotional center and you will have certain emotion with that thought. It also causes release of different transmitters, and they excite or inhibit the other center in the brain. These centers affect the peripheral nervous system, hormones and immune system in the body. Every thought has some effect on your feelings, your physiology and biochemistry in your body.

If the thought is short and with no significant emotions with it, the effects are minimal. But when you have negative thoughts all day long, and especially when they are with lots of strong emotions, then the effect become significant. These negative thoughts over time can make you emotionally and physically ill. This is way our unconscious mind and our beliefs are so important, because they are affecting our body most of the time, even during sleep.

For example, there are some people worried about everything, from safety of their children in school to their relationship, health, or financial matters. These people end up with anxiety and panic attacks. The thought with its feeling makes our attitude. Our attitude can directly affect the outcome of your health and the treatment you receive. The positive attitude "I will be better" or "I will heal" will affect your body positively. But a negative attitude such as "I will have this pain forever" or "This pain will not go away," will affect the body negatively.

Remember that your thoughts can become a self-fulfilling prophecy. Our unconscious and conscious mind controls the body.

Effect of Our Thoughts on Genes Expression

Human genome is the complete set of genetic instruction, which contains all the information for growth and development as a human. These instructions, or genome, are made from DNA (Deoxyribonucleic acid). Human genome has 3.2 billion of pair of DNA. DNA is made up four nucleotides base; adenine, cytosine, guanine and thymine or in short A, C, G and T. The order of these nucleosides subunits makes the DNA code. DNA has double helix shape.

Each single strand of DNA collided in one of the 46 human chromosomes (23 pair) which are located in cell nucleus. Our body consists of one hundred trillion cells. The gene is a segment of DNA and is the basic physical code of hereditary. Humans have about 20,000 to 25,000 gens. (Average 23,000)

Gene expression is the process by which the genetic instruction is converted to functional products, such as proteins. Thousands of these gene expressions inside each cell determine cell's function. The genes don't have always ultimate power over emotional and physical health and well-being. We are not doomed to our genes. We can affect the gene expression by our thoughts and behavior.

These days, there is a lot of talk about genes for different emotional and physical illness, or even for bad habits and addiction. Only a very small percentage of the genes for certain diseases can express themselves one hundred percent. Most of the time, the genes only predispose the person to a certain illness, then the thoughts, behavior and environment will determine the final result.

Therefore, we are not the victim of our genome. We do have a choice and we can change the final result of what our genome is going to bring to our life. For example, they studied the identical twins that grew up in different environments, compared with non-identical twins who grow up in the same environment.

The first group (identical twins) had more different active and non-active genes than non-identical twins who grew up in the same environment. This finding shows the effect of the environment on the genes. The environment affects the person's thoughts, beliefs, habits and behavior. When individuals grow up in different environment, they think, feel and respond differently. There could be other factors in each environment that affect the gene expression, but I think the main factor is the thoughts and behavior.

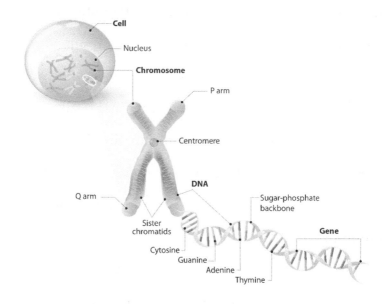

Epigenetic studies show that genes are not your destiny. Your thoughts and behavior will affect the gene expression. If somebody has the gene for an illness, it is not written in stone that he/she for sure will come up with that illness. With our thoughts and behaviors, we can change our destiny. We can go through our whole life and the effects of some of our genes never show up.

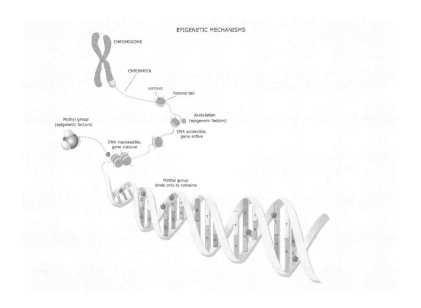

For example, if you have a history of diabetes or heart disease in your family, if you think about it all the time and are fearful about it, your chance of becoming diabetic or having heart disease increases, especially if you believe (at an unconscious level) that you are going to become sick.

Instead, it is better to have thoughts like, *I will be healthy, I will have a long life, I am going to have a healthy heart.* These positive thoughts and beliefs give you hope and determination to have a healthy life style and do the necessary prevention. With positive thinking, not only diabetes and the heart disease may not show up in your own life, but you'll also reduce the chance of these illnesses in the next generations.

When you think health, happiness, and healing, these thoughts become your beliefs and manifest in your body.

How the Brain Regulates the Body

In the first section of this chapter, we discussed that our thoughts and beliefs affect our body, health and healing. I have no doubt that my thoughts affect my health, therefore, I carefully choose my thoughts.

How do our thoughts and beliefs affect our body? Our thoughts make some changes in our brain's chemistry, physiology, and structure. These activities send different signals to the body through the nervous system, endocrine and immune system.

These are the ways the brain regulate the body. I describe each system briefly. Knowing these systems will help you to understand and appreciate that your thoughts really affect your body through changes in your brain. The brain is in constant communication with different organs in your body.

From unconscious activities such as breathing and heart rate to moving or talking are under control of your brain. Changes in physiology and chemistry in the body send feedback to the brain. The brain receives the feedback and readjusts to keep the body in a hemostasis.

Nervous System

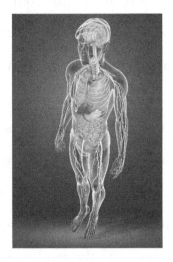

How does the brain receive and send information from and to the body and the world? The crown of the skull (cranium) houses the brain, protects it from harm and separates it from the outside world. The brain connects to the body and outside world through the peripheral nervous system. (Central nervous system consists of the brain and the spinal cord).

The peripheral nervous system consists of the nerves that branch out of the brain and spinal cord, which are called **cranial and spinal nerves**. These nerves send information to and from the brain and the spinal cord. The sensory nerves send signals from the receptors all over the body to the brain for the processing. The brain receives information from the outside world through the sensory organs.

The brain, after collecting and interpreting data, sends a response to the body through motor nerves. There are two kinds of motor nerves. First is the **voluntary motor nerves** (or **somatic**) that are under conscious control. For example; the nerves carry the sending signals to skeletal muscle to move. The second part is the **autonomic or involuntary** motor nerves, which carry the unconscious responses from the brain to different parts of the body, like the heart. The brain regulates the vital, everyday function of the body through the autonomic nervous system.

The autonomic nervous system has two divisions; the **sympathetic** and **parasympathetic** branch. The sympathetic branch is the more wakefulness and alert side and parasympathetic is the calmer side. The knowledge about the sympathetic and parasympathetic nervous system is important for understanding the effect of different thoughts on the body. At times of stress, the sympathetic division becomes activated and the heart rate and blood pressure go up.

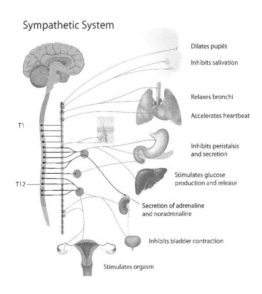

Sympathetic System

Dilates pupils

Inhibits salivation

Relaxes bronchi

Accelerates heartbeat

Inhibits peristalsis and secretion

Stimulates glucose production and release

Secretion of adrenaline and noradrenaline

Inhibits bladder contraction

Stimulates orgasm

T1

T12

The sympathetic nervous system also activates with fear and excitement. When you See something you are afraid of activates your sympathetic nervous system.

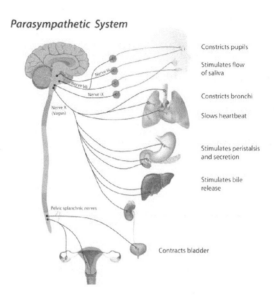

Parasympathetic System

The parasympathetic nervous system is more involved in the relaxation mode. It quiets and relaxes the body. Meditation that activates the parasympathetic division, the heart rate and blood pressure drops (also called relaxation response).

Both these systems are equally important for the safety and balance of the body. You need an active sympathetic system at times of danger. And after the danger passes, you need the parasympathetic system to return the body to the calm state. In chronic stress, the sympathetic system is activated most of the time and keeps the body in an alert state. I will discuss in chapter 5 how to activate the parasympathetic system for returning the body and mind to a calmer state.

Endocrine System

The endocrine system works with the nervous system to regulate the body. The endocrine system includes organs that produce hormones. The hypothalamus is the link between the brain and endocrine system. The hypothalamus releases hormones directly to the blood and also, hypothalamus controls the pituitary gland.

The pituitary gland releases various hormones that control the other glands throughout the body.

The endocrine organs, when releasing hormones, regulate the different organs' functions. The circulating hormones also have an effect on the brain and the behavior.

Our thoughts affect the endocrine system and make it to release hormones that regulate many functions such as metabolism and growth. Stress activates the hypothalamic-pituitary-adrenal (HPA) axis. As a result, the adrenal gland produces cortisol, which affects different parts of the body.

HORMONES

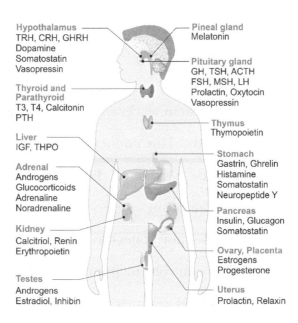

Hypothalamus
TRH, CRH, GHRH
Dopamine
Somatostatin
Vasopressin

Pineal gland
Melatonin

Pituitary gland
GH, TSH, ACTH
FSH, MSH, LH
Prolactin, Oxytocin
Vasopressin

Thyroid and
Parathyroid
T3, T4, Calcitonin
PTH

Thymus
Thymopoietin

Liver
IGF, THPO

Stomach
Gastrin, Ghrelin
Histamine
Somatostatin
Neuropeptide Y

Adrenal
Androgens
Glucocorticoids
Adrenaline
Noradrenaline

Pancreas
Insulin, Glucagon
Somatostatin

Kidney
Calcitriol, Renin
Erythropoietin

Ovary, Placenta
Estrogens
Progesterone

Testes
Androgens
Estradiol, Inhibin

Uterus
Prolactin, Relaxin

The Immune System

The immune system includes all the organs related to immunity in the body. The brain and the immune system communicate with each other. The mental state can affect the immune system. The study of connection between the nervous system and the immune system is called **psychoneuroimmunology.**

Changes in the brain cause changes in the immune system. The changes in hypothalamus affect the immune system response, for example, in patients with tumor and allergies. Thoughts can produce changes in the immune system. An example of how your state of mind affects the immune system can be seen in people with depression.

There is evidence that depression impairs the immune system and increases the risk of illness. Depressed individuals have a reduction in the activity of natural killer cells (these blood cells are necessary for fighting and killing cancer cells).

The communication between the brain and immune system works both way.

Immune system activities influence the brain. When the immune system produces antibodies to fight infection, we can see changes in neuronal activities in different parts of the brain, such as the hypothalamus. The brain will be notified of what is happening in the immune system.

Immune conditioning is a strong evidence of the interaction of the mind and immune system. The immune system can respond to a psychological stimulus such as taste or smell associated with immunosuppressive drugs the same way it would respond to drugs. In the first stage of experiment, the patient would receive the special smells while receiving the immunosuppressive drug.

In the second stage, the patient would receive the same smell with a much lower dose of the drug. The response in the second stage was similar to the first stage. The sense of smell in the brain triggers the same response in the patient.

The immunosuppressive drugs have significant side effects. Some patients need to use a high dose of immunosuppressive drugs for a long time possible their whole life. The immune conditioning has been used to reduce the dosage of these drugs.

IMMUNE SYSTEM

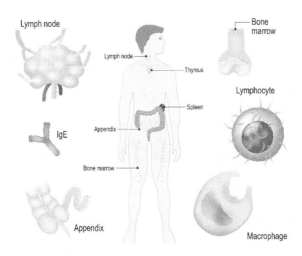

How Our Thoughts and Feelings Affect Weight Loss

You can lose weight by changing your thoughts and behavior. Feeling bad about your body and yourself will not help in losing weight. There is usually a thought pattern of overeating. Emotional eating is a problem for many people; they eat to cool down their emotions.

The neuronal network, which has been formed in the brain, will be activated every time they are stressed and they go for the food. If they change their thoughts from food and focus on something else, it gives them time to think and stop this vicious loop.

You can find healthier ways to deal with your emotions and stop emotional eating. Depression is linked to being overweight. Positive thinking has a significant role in losing weight. Positive thoughts are empowering and increase energy level. Keep the ideal image of the body you would like to have and work toward it.

If you think negatively, you will have a more difficult time to lose weight. When you think negatively, you do not have the necessary motivation and stamina to change your habit. The negative thoughts may lead to self-defeating behavior such as changing your plan of eating healthy, overeating and skipping exercise.

The State of Mind and the Treatment Outcome

Your state of mind affects your healing. Your state of mind or attitude is very powerful. Positive beliefs like "I will get better," "I will recover," "This medication will help me," or "I will come out of the surgery" will positively affect the treatment outcome. The effect of the state of mind on healing has been shown in different studies. The belief that something will help can actually help. This positive attitude helps your healing in several ways.

- You will be more hopeful, and as the result more relaxed and less stressed and fearful. When you are relaxed, your body heals faster.
- Because you think that the treatment will help you, you follow the treatment protocol more carefully.
- The positive outlook affects your perception, you see more positive things in your life than negative. The more positive things you see in your life, the more grateful and happy you are.

Life Purpose Affects Health and Longevity

Your purpose in life is the central point of your life. Keep your purpose in front of you when you are ill. Cherish your vision and dreams; one day, you will enter that world. When you imagine your dreams vividly and long enough without too much interruption, your brain structure will change. Your vision network becomes more interconnected and stronger. As a result, you will come up with ideas and ways to achieve that goal. When this idea becomes mixed with emotion that means the emotional center in the brain gets activated, make yourself to take the necessary action. Emotion causes motion and action. When you have an idea with emotion, you are motivated and you take necessary action and you will produce results.

If you keep your focus on your health and healing, your body will transform. If you keep beautiful and lovely thoughts in your mind, one day, they will become your reality. Think of the organs in your body as they are healthy and working perfectly. Imagine a long, happy, healthy life.

If you want to have a beautiful, healthy body, you need to have beautiful, healthy thoughts and vision. Having a purpose in life, especially during the healing process, is important because most diseases are discouraging and frustrating. Our vision keeps our mind and body alive.

It is very essential that you don't let discouraging circumstances, disease, or pain change your vision and purpose. People who have a purpose have a happier, calmer, and longer life. When you have a purpose in life, you are stronger and have more of a chance to survive.

Older people who have a purpose in their lives and are looking forward to achieving something usually live longer.

The Power of Thoughts on Life

As I discussed earlier in this chapter, our thoughts affect our health and healing directly through the connection of our brain to the body. I explained how this happens through nervous, endocrine and immune systems. Our thoughts also affect our happiness, health and healing through our choices and behavior. When we keep a thought long enough in our mind and dwell on it, we start talking and acting based on that thought.

As Emerson said, *"the ancestor of every action is a thought."* This is why it is so important what kind of thoughts we keep running in our minds most of the time. Any thought or idea can come to our mind at any moment, but we have the choice to keep thinking about that thought or idea. A thought is just a thought; it could be real or not, positive or negative, useful or useless.

It does not mean that because we had such a thought, we are a good or bad person. But we are responsible for examining that thought and deciding to keep dwelling on it, talking about it or take any action. This needs discipline and awareness. It is much easier to blame than to find out the real cause of the problem.

One reason we don't learn from our mistakes and instead, repeat them is because we do not think hard enough to find out the real problem. We may even have wrong conclusions of our experiences. Thoughts affect everything in your life. Having a healthy life and being happy is not separate from your whole life as a human being.

The other areas of life, such as family, relationships, finances, and profession, will affect your health and healing. For example, if we make decisions that affect our relationship and family negatively, it will cause stress that can affect our health mentally, emotionally and physically.

When you keep your mind and brain healthy and make wise decisions, it will affect your happiness, and you will have a happier life. Happiness is not something that you make or find. Happiness comes from your thoughts and actions. Our health, happiness and healing are related to the rest of your lives.

Balance in life is essential for having a successful and fulfilling life. You can achieve this balance in your life with a balanced and organized mind. You need to control your thoughts and keep them in the right direction as much as possible.

Tip: Try to be more aware and make conscious choices rather than habitual and unconscious ones.

In summary, I believe that, without question, our thoughts make us. If you want to have a good and healthy life, guard your thoughts and choose positive ones.

We are all the master of our thoughts. We can choose our thoughts. If a thought comes to mind and is not empowering, simply say, "Cancel," and take your attention away from that thought, and then choose the thought you want.

Choose the thoughts you want from the stream of positive, loving, healthy, and peaceful thoughts. Your thoughts will affect your life and your body. In any situation, thoughts of love, joy, and peace must be your top priority. If your thoughts are not thoughts of joy, peace, and love, you need to stop and find a couple of minutes for yourself and bring those thoughts back.

Chapter Four
Positive and Happy Thoughts

"If you realized how powerful your thoughts are,

you would never think negative thoughts."

—Peace Pilgrim

Positive Beliefs and Positive Thinking

It is important to know the difference between thoughts and beliefs.

Thoughts are in the conscious mind. You have thousands of them going through your mind daily. Your thought will change as soon as you start thinking or focus on something else. Thoughts are part of the working memory. Someone said that *ideas are like fish, they slip away quickly.*

The reason is that you keep thoughts as long as you are thinking and concentrating on them. As soon as you pay attention to something else, that idea is gone unless it has been written down or remember at later time. If you want to think positively most of the day, you actively need to focus on the positive; otherwise your thoughts revert back to negative as soon as you focus on the negative.

When you think about something positive, the content of your consciousness is positive. The negative content of your consciousness will change with your thought process.

A belief is a thought that you accept as true. Your beliefs are in your unconscious mind and they run your life 24 hours a day. Your beliefs will not change like thoughts from one moment to the next moment. The beliefs are a part of the structure of the brain. If the same thought is repeated and is accepted by the subconscious mind as truth, then that thought becomes your new belief.

If a person has another belief that is contradictory to the new thought, the new thought will be rejected and does not become part of long-term memory. The structure of the brain will not change and the person will be stuck with her/his own original belief. Your beliefs have power over your life, because you act based on those beliefs.

That is the reason why the beliefs are so powerful. Your beliefs are part of your unconscious mind and they will affect your decisions and actions. Most of us without awareness let them run our lives. We can change this, by becoming more aware and act differently.

This can become possible if we are present in the moment, paying attention and choosing differently. We can also change the old belief with a new belief. It takes time and effort, but we are able to do that.

Positive Thinking

Positive thinking is expecting good and favorable results in life. When you think positively, you approach life's challenges with a positive outlook. It does not mean you ignore the bad things; instead, you try to see the best and make the most of a potentially bad situation. **The human brain can do anything if it thinks it can do it. Our brain learns from the thoughts in our mind and starts looking for what we have been thinking**.

Positive thinking can help you in more ways than you may realize. When you think positively, you will not allow your mind to entertain negative thoughts.

The health benefits of positive thinking have shown in multiple studies. There is a link between positive thinking, emotional and physical health.

According to the Mayo Clinic, positive thinking has health benefits, such as better emotional health, a lower rate of depression, less stress, a lower rate of death related to cardiovascular disease, and longer life. Positive thinking is also important for having a healthy brain.

The positive thoughts have healing power. The idea that with positive thoughts you can help yourself heal and have a longer life, almost seems too good to be true.

However, I can assure you, I have experienced and witnessed the health benefits that positive thinking can bring to us. The more you focus on positive things in your life, the more likely you will enjoy a sense of well-being in your life.

As James Allen said in his book, As a man Thinketh, *"Good thoughts bring good results; bad thoughts bring bad results."*

If you want to have a healthy body, you need to have healthy and positive thoughts. The body itself has a marvelous self-healing system, but negative thoughts can interfere with this system. Positive thinking affects your health in a positive way. As we discussed in last chapter, our thoughts affect our body through the peripheral nervous system, endocrine and immune system. The positive thoughts affect these systems positively. Think about each organ of your body as it is healthy and working perfectly.

The thoughts inside your mind will one day manifest outwardly in your life. The people who think positively have stronger immune systems. The immune system produces more helper T cells, (A Type of T cells that provides help to other cells in the immune system) therefore it can fights infection and cancers better.

Positive thinking can help reduce symptoms. This means if you have a headache or back pain, if you think positively, it will help you to feel less pain. If you think that you are feeling differently, you will feel differently. If you think healthy and strong, you will feel healthy and strong. Your thoughts can make you instantly feel happy or sad, calm or anxious.

The positive thoughts lead to corresponding emotions and actions that affect your life positively. If you think positively about your health and healing, you will change how you feel and act about your health. We can decide what to think and therefore we have control over our life, including our health and healing.

It is especially important to keep positive thoughts when you have a sick family member. When you see a family member with an illness, it affects your thoughts, and you may start thinking, *"will it happen to me, too?"* But the key here is to change your thoughts and say, *"with my healthy thoughts and behavior, I will be healthy."*

When we are sick, different negative thoughts will come to our mind. We should change them to positive ones. We need to expect the best result from our tests and treatment. Focus on the good results, even the smallest of improvements.

Positive Beliefs

As the late Dr. Wayne Dyer once said, *"you attract not what you want, but what you are."*

What you are is your beliefs in your unconscious mind and they are working all the time. But **what you want** is in your mind as long as you are thinking about it, and can change before affect your decision and behavior and give any result.

You attract things to you that are deeply rooted in your unconsciousness. What you believe becomes your reality. Your underlying beliefs influence medical treatments. The limiting and negative beliefs about your health and healing affect your health and healing negatively.

For example, if you heard a negative belief about a specific disease and treatment in childhood, it will influence your healing. Most of these negative and harmful beliefs are not true. You have got these beliefs from the information you have received and accepted without any question since childhood.

If you believe, "my family has diabetes; I will get diabetes by this age," unfortunately, this negative belief increases your risk of diabetes. If you believe, "I have bad genes," this will affect your healing. When you change your beliefs about your health and healing, you can change the gene's expression.

You can activate the good genes and inactivate the ones that are bad for your health. Your genes do not determine the final results. They may predispose you to a disease or a condition, but you have the ultimate say with your thoughts, beliefs and behavior.

You did not have these beliefs. You have learned all these negative beliefs. You have a choice and you can change these beliefs to true and positive ones. As a result, you will change your health, healing and life's outcome. You can have a life that is very different from your parents, family and the life you lived so far. You can have a longer life than your parents.

As TD Jakes said, *"don't let your history become your destiny."*

Positive beliefs have a positive influence on health and healing. If you have beliefs like, *"I am strong. I will heal fast, and the treatment will help"* It can positively affect your healing. In my own practice, I've had patients who've been depressed and had negative beliefs about their back pain. They heard and believed they had to live with this back pain, and unfortunately, many continued to have back pain even after a successful surgery. This does not need to be in the case in your life.

Your belief system can be derived from your culture, religion, and family. You hear and learn different beliefs from child hood and usually accept them as truth. These beliefs will affect your health and healing for the rest of your life. These beliefs could be positive or negative. Many studies have shown the beneficial effect of a positive belief on a variety of illnesses.

The placebo affect demonstrates the power of your beliefs on healing. For example, the placebo effect has been shown in medications. When sugar pills were given to a group of people and were told these medications will help. When they believed these are medication, they actually worked like real medication for those people.

Changing your underlying beliefs and inner voices can be difficult, but if you become aware of these negative beliefs, with effort, you can replace them with empowering beliefs that can change your life.

Beliefs affect how the genes are expressed. Studies on human genes and genetic makeup of our DNA are very complex. Prediction of a specific illness based on the genome is not as simplistic as once thought and manifestation of a gene is affected by different factors, including your beliefs and thoughts.

If a person has a serious illness such as cancer, instead of fear and believing of all bad things that he or she has heard, instead, they should try to believe that "*I am going to heal*" without having any doubt. The brain cannot do what it needs to do effectively when there is doubt.

The doubt interferes with the brain work. The doubt is activation of another network in the brain that affects the main positive belief network, therefore, the positive belief will not have all its effect on the mind, body, emotions and behavior. Doubt reduces the strength of the belief.

Happy Thoughts

"Happiness does not depend on who you are or what you have; it depends solely on what you think."

-Dale Carnegie

Happy and joyful thoughts are associated with positive physiological and chemical changes in the body. Happy thoughts make you calmer, and you feel more in control.

What is happiness? Happiness is a state that is associated with experiencing joy, contentment, positive well-being, and calmness. It is a feeling of warmth and richness in life and wanting to live.

Research on the human brain has showed several regions related to happiness. They include the hypothalamus and nucleus accumbens. The neurotransmitter dopamine, which releases in these centers, is associated with an increase in the sense of pleasure. Based on modern neuroscience, we know that positive emotions, such as happiness, enthusiasm and compassion, can be trained.

We can learn to be happier. Our brain structure will change in a way that we can become happy easier and faster, our happiness lasts longer, and also, we can have higher levels of happiness. This will happen as the result of changes in the pattern of neuronal activation by making different and new neuronal connections in the brain.

So, how can this information can help you? The good news is that you can learn to be happy like learning any other skills. If you were unhappy until now, you have the choice and ability to be happy from this moment on. You do not need to wait until your life conditions change to be happy.

You can be happy and at the same time, vigorously work to make necessary changes in your life. Life is a journey; you do not have to wait to be happy later. If you are not happy now and continue the same thought process, you may not be happy in the future. If you become happy for achieving your goal, it may last only for a short time.

Practice being happy now, and your brain learns this pattern to be happy with what you have. When you achieve your goals and conditions of your life, you will be even happier.

Christian D. Larson in the JUST BE GLAD wrote: *"Do not think that happiness must keep its distance so long as you have so much to pass through. The more you have to pass through, the more you need your happiness. It is the shining countenance that never turns back; it is the glad heart that finds strength to go on;*

it is the mind with the most sunshine that can see the most clearly where to go and how to act that the goal in view may be gained."

How does happiness affect the body?

"Happiness is the highest form of health."

—Dalai Lama

Happy thoughts build a happy body. Happy people live longer and have less cancer and cardiovascular disease than unhappy people. As Dr. Lissa Rankin said in her book, Mind Over Medicine, *"Happiness is a preventative medicine."* When you are sick, your attention usually is on the signs and symptoms of the disease, like pain, fever, or nausea. By simply changing your thoughts to a happy, calm situation, you can feel better.

For example, if you have nausea, try to change your thoughts from feeling nauseous to something enjoyable, like scenery or fresh air. These thoughts can help you to feel better. James Allen wrote nicely: *"There is no physician like a cheerful thought for dissipating the ills of the body."*

There are people who question how they can be happy while having so many problems in their lives. The answer is that happiness comes from inside. Happiness is a sense of well-being, a sense that you have the ability to deal with life challenges. When you are happy, your body responds with good health. Everybody has challenges and obstacles in their lives. When you are happy, you will be better at handling these situations and circumstances.

When you are happy, you have more energy and stamina. You feel more in control; you don't feel overwhelmed. All these feelings reduce stress levels and allow your body to heal.

Our level of happiness really can impact the level of our health. Happy people recover faster than unhappy people. For example, in a study of the patients who had the same severity of head injury, the patients who were happy prior to the head injury recovered faster, compared to the people who were depressed prior to the head injury.

Happiness is also correlated with longevity. In the study of nuns, the researchers found out the importance of relationship between happiness and longevity. In this group of nuns most of their lifestyle variables were the same. The researchers found that at the age of 85 years old, 90 percent of the most cheerful nuns were still alive, but only 34 percent of the least cheerful nuns lived to this age.

Remember this: if you are happier, not only would you enjoy your life, but you will also be healthier and live longer. Happiness also affects the brain's function. **It has been shown that when we are happy, we make fewer mistakes.** We are also more creative and have fewer errors, which are influenced by our habits.

Depression

When I talk about depression, it hits me, and I sometimes get a tear in my eye because it reminds me of relatives and many other people I know with depression. Some of them had tragic consequences. Depression affects all aspects of life. It affects not only the body but also family, work, and finances.

Depression is a disease and affects too many people. In the United States, 2 to 3 percent of the population suffers from severe depression. Depression can affect children as young as five years old.

Individuals with depression usually experience four or five of the following symptoms daily, for more than two weeks.

- Depressed mood
- Loss of interest or pleasure
- Fatigue and loss of energy
- Changes to appetite and sleep patterns
- Social withdrawal
- Suicidal thoughts
- Feeling of hopelessness
- Feeling of emptiness
- Impaired concentration and memory
- Crying spells without specific reason

What are the changes in the brain in the patients with depression? They may have an imbalance of the neurotransmitters in the brain, such as serotonin, dopamine, or norepinephrine. Depression involves the cerebral cortex, amygdala, hippocampus, hypothalamus, and other areas of the brain.

Depression can cause shrinkage of the hippocampus (the region of the brain that regulates stress), and that in turn affects the ability to regulate stress. Depressed people get stressed faster and easier.

Depression also affects the frontal lobe, which is the place for reasoning, and decreases rational thinking over the emotional limbic system.

Although heredity plays a role in developing depression, it is largely environmental and socioeconomic. People with a serious illness or life changes such as divorce or loss of a loved one may experience depression.

How Depression Affects the Body

"I have decided to be happy because it good for my health."

- Voltaire

Unhappy people are more likely to get sick from diseases like cancer, heart disease, and pain disorders. For example, most of the patients I see who have chronic pain and fibromyalgia suffer from depression.

The Harvard Happiness Study, one of the longest studies in happiness, which spanned over several decades, showed that individuals who were unhappy had more chronic illnesses and died sooner.

A study of American men showed that depressed men developed cancer twice as often in later years, compared to non-depressed men.

Depressed people are not motivated and usually do not have a healthy behavior, which also affects their emotional and physical health. Depression increases the risk of conditions like addiction and suicide, which in turn increase the risks of diseases and death. Depressed people usually do not look after themselves; they do not get enough sleep, have a proper diet, or exercise. These healthy life styles such as proper sleep, diet and exercise are necessary for having a healthy body.

The good news is that people with depression can be healed and become happy again.

Individuals with depression should seek professional help. Depression is a disease and should be treated. There is no reason to hide depression. Depression not only affects the life of the patient, but also affects the life of other family members and especially children. **The**

treatment of depression is easier if it starts early. The sooner depression is treated, the less adverse effects it has on the body and mind.

The people around the person with depression should encourage he/she to start the treatment as soon as possible. The research has shown a strong link between depression and suicide. As the depression deepens and takes over the brain and mind, the pain becomes overwhelming.

The deep despair and chemical changes in the brain can lead to the brain starting to find a way to end the pain. At this point, the suicidal thoughts come to mind. Patients with depression are also suffering from thoughts of hopelessness and helplessness which also can add to the suicidal thoughts.

The depression is treatable and suicide is preventable. The patients with depression and their families should get any help which is available. If the family notices any sign of suicidal thoughts in the patient with depression, they should not leave them alone. The family should get help as soon as possible.

The approach to treatment of depression will vary from person to person. There are many sources available for helping and treating patients with depression. I have outlined some suggestions for helping patients with depression, but I strongly suggest to get the appropriate help you need. You don't have to live with depression. Remember that you are not the depression. You are a person that has depression. Never own the depression. You were a happy person one time.

There are different reasons for depression. Some people may have genes that predispose them to depression, but in the happy and calm environment, those genes may never express themselves in an entire life time. Some of the reasons for depression are serious illness, lost loved one, or divorce. But a person who has gotten depressed for any reason, there is hope to become happy again.

Anyone with depression should start doing whatever they can do to overcome the depression. When a person is depressed, they cannot think as clearly as when he/she is happy and may make decisions that could make the situation even worse!

If you are depressed, the healing starts with you. Stop self-pity and nurturing the depression. It is better to get rid of the depression and get your joy back again than manage the depression. You deserve to have a life full of joy.

"You have no cause for anything but gratitude and joy."

-Buddha

Some Suggestions

- Socialize and talk to family and friends (patients with depression usually are withdrawn from family and friends). When you talk to others about your depression, you start feeling less overwhelmed and see the depression as something which has affected you, rather than you owning it. You can feel like more of an observer that enables you to control the depression.

- Exercise helps elevate the mood. Exercise activates the left prefrontal cortex. By activating the left prefrontal cortex, that is the rational center, the patient will think more rationally. Activation of the left prefrontal cortex also makes the person happier (people with depression are usually less active.)

- Proper diets; patients with depression usually do not have a proper diet. There is evidence that a diet rich in fruit and vegetables is related to positive mood and more happiness. Omega 3, vitamin D and B vitamins (especially vitamin B12, B6 and folate) will help depression.

- Proper sleep is very important for having a good mood. Most of the patients with depression do not have good quality sleep.

- Cognitive therapy is one of the treatments for depression. In this treatment, the patient will start referring to depression in a more positive way. It increases the cognitive function of the brain and decreases the emotional part. As the result, the person starts thinking more rationally and less emotionally.

- Every day, as soon as you wake up in the morning, say, "I want to feel good. I want to be happy. I choose to be happy." Then do the things that make you happy. In a matter of time, your mood will improve and you will be happier.

- Patients with depression may need to get antidepressant medication initially if other therapies are not enough. But treating depression with antidepressant medication alone is not enough. You need medication to help you to get rid of depression, while you are thinking and behaving in new ways and rewire your brain. You can become a happy person again and not need any medication. The medications help to increase several neurotransmitters in your brain to improve your mood. You can do the same with changing your thinking and behavior like happy people do.

People with depression need to look into their life and ask what can be the cause of their depression. They must attempt to change the stressful situations. They also need to change themselves from the inside and the way they perceive the outside world. There are going to be challenges in almost everyone's life, but there is no need to become depressed.

You may become sad for some time, that is one of our primary emotions, and there is nothing wrong with it. But the problem starts when you let this sadness turn into depression. In history, we read that when somebody in a tribe would lose a loved one, they were allowed to wear black clothes and mourn only for a special period of time. After that period of time they would have to change to regular clothes and life.

If we think about it, there is good wisdom in it. We need to do the same thing in any situation that has caused us sadness. After an initial period of sadness, we need to let it go, forgive, change our response and start a new life. We should not let it turns into depression and cause changes in our brain.

There is always a way if you look hard enough. There is always hope. There is always help. As long as you are alive, there is a way! If you feel hopeless, you need to change your thinking and look harder. There is hope. You just need to keep looking for it.

Optimistic Thoughts

Are optimistic people healthier and do they live longer than pessimistic people? The answer is yes. Many studies have shown that the optimistic people are emotionally and physically healthier and live longer than pessimistic people. Pessimists are more likely to become depressed and get sick.

Hope helps healing. The feeling of hopefulness affects whether we stay healthy, get sick or recover from illness. When you have a sickness, you may see the doctor and you have some tests. As you are waiting for the results, you should think, *"the results are going to be good."*

Expect the best of medication. Expect the best of surgery.

Also, it is important to remember, when you expect the best from your treatment, you believe what you are hoping for is actually going to happen. You do not entertain any doubt or make back up plans in a case it did not work.

When the Harvard Happiness Study reviewed optimism and pessimism, researchers found that optimistic individuals recovered faster and lived longer.

The pessimists got sick younger, had more severe illnesses, and recovered less quickly.

Some patients, as soon as they hear the diagnosis of a serious illness like cancer, lose hope and think that the disease will eventually kill them. So, they give up.

In a situation like this, losing hope has many negative consequences. It affects your immune system, causes stress, and increases depression. Unfortunately, when patients lose hope, they do not put all their effort into their treatment. Losing hope makes them think the treatment will not work. Therefore, be hopeful all the time, despite negative results or temporary setbacks. You must stay hopeful.

Hope keeps people alive! It gets them out of a difficult situation and helps them to heal. They will have stronger immune systems. Their bodies fight infection and disease better. Hopeful thinking says, *"Disease is temporary, and the situation will turn around."* Say to yourself, "I will heal, this will pass."

In my own practice, I had a patient with alcoholism who had fallen twice after getting hit by a car. I had removed a blood clot from over his brain. After the second surgery, he and I talked about hope.

He shared with me part of his life. He said his wife left him, and he was alone. He did not think anyone would marry him. I told him if he had hope and stopped drinking, his life would change; he could marry again and could even have a family.

I saw him several months later. He said that he has stopped drinking, got a job and was going to start a family.

That is the result of hope. The state of hopelessness and helplessness is one of the worst situations to find yourself; you may end up in a tragic situation like suicide.

There are many stories about how hope saves people. It has been reported how some people who had been severely injured, even bleeding, stayed alive while they waited for a loved one to arrive.

"However bad life may seem, there is always something you can do and succeed at. While there's life, there is hope."

—Stephen Hawking

Imagination

"If you form a picture in your mind of what you would like to be, and keep and hold that picture long enough, you will soon become as you have been thinking."

-William James

To feel positive and be happy, imagine what you want to happen. It has been shown that imagination affects the neurons like we are really doing what we are imagining. During imagination, the neurons which we are using make new connections.

When you imagine, the structure of your brain will change. These changes are in the direction you want your life to go. When these changes happen in your brain, you will see your life as you imagined, you will act in this new way and your wish will be fulfilled.

That is so important when you are ill; do not visualize your current circumstances. You want to imagine you are healed or healing. If you can imagine that you are already healed, it will have a stronger effect on your brain and as a result, on your body. It is very important that you believe what you visualize will happen.

Imagination is the workshop of the mind.

This is your workshop and you have all tools you need to make anything you want. Make the things you want and love. Tesla invented many of his inventions in his mind. Your vision needs to be bigger than your current circumstances. You may have, for example, an infection in your body, you have pain, fever, you are in the hospital and you are receiving intravenous antibiotics.

You need to imagine that fever and pain is gone. The antibiotics and your immune system are getting rid of infection and your organs are functioning normally. When you imagine a healthy body, it will affect the gene expression and restructure your body the way you imagined. Imagine the good result of the test and the good things that you want to happen in the future.

I ask my patients in the hospital, "What would you like to do when you go home?" The answers are different. For example, "Travel," "See my grandchildren," "Celebrate the holidays," or just simply, "Be at home." Then I will tell them, "Visualize you already there, even when you are lying down in bed here."

I also tell patients in the intensive care unit, "You are here in ICU, but you can be as happy or as miserable as you want to be. It depends on your thoughts. When you visualize happiness, you will heal faster and you will be happy instead of suffering."

When you imagine, do it with emotion. The more feeling and emotion with imagination, the better it will affect you. Take time to remember the fun times you had in the past. Think about scenery or going somewhere exciting, and try to duplicate the feelings you have at those moments.

Watch Happy and Healthy Programs

Our thoughts form in our brain as the result of electrical and chemical activities of neuronal networks. These networks activate as the result of the internal and external stimuli. The external stimuli are the information the brain receives from the outside world through our sensory organs, such as eyes and ears.

We can control which neurons are activated by choosing what we watch, hear, our environment and people around us. It is much easier to think about something happy when you are watching something happy and funny. Watching happy and healthy programs will help you to more easily visualize the good results. After watching an inspiring program or movie, those pictures will be in your mind.

Also, watch comedies; they make you happier and cause you to think about funny things. If you visualize joyful images, it will energize you. Watch the happy ending story of people who were healed. Do not read or watch negative news about the bad result. When you are sick, your body is already under a lot of stress; do not add more stress to it. Instead, listen to calming music, nature sounds, or what makes you calm and happy.

When you have an emotional or physical illness, avoid watching negative news and programs. Viewing negative news and programs affects your thoughts, and you'll start feeling bad.

Focus on What You Want

What you focus on will expand. If you focus on what you want and what you love, those thoughts will expand in your mind. These thoughts would activate the other nerve cells, and your thoughts will expand.

Positive thinking is focusing on what you want and thinking about what you love. It will bring you happiness. When you focus on what you want, you'll find a way to get those things. You cannot find a way to get the things you want by thinking about the things you don't want.

If you think about the things you want, you will find a way. That's how you solve the problem. You solve it because you focus strongly on the solution instead.

Stop Dwelling on Negative Thoughts

If negative thoughts such as anger, frustration, loneliness, and fear come to your mind, try not to rehearse them in your mind. Instead, try to get them out of your mind. If you rehearse a negative thought in your mind over and over, it becomes magnified and you feel even worse.

You can become more upset than you were originally. There are ways that can help you to stop dwelling on negative thoughts and refocus on positive thoughts. Such as;

- Choose a different thought.
- By distracting yourself.
- Imagine you are doing something pleasant in your mind.
- Talk to a positive and happy person.
- Do something that makes you happy and calm. For example go for walk or have a cup of tea.

Negative beliefs and thoughts affect the body's natural self-repair mechanism and predispose the body to disease. Keeping your mind clear of negative thoughts is very important when you are in the healing process.

When we have an illness, our body is already under stress. Negative thoughts such as anger, fear, and frustration cause more stress, and stress affects the body's natural healing. Negative thoughts and feelings also affect the brain and turn off the motivation circuit in the brain. We lose our motivation, at the time we need motivation to work on our healing.

Joy, appreciation, and love reverse the effects of negative thoughts and feelings.

Love

Love is the most positive feeling and has been talked about in all religions and cultures. Love is essential for healing. When you love yourself, you can share this love with others. Love reduces stress. Many people today think they do not deserve love. They may have heard these thoughts during childhood. These thoughts often come from the criticism of people around us. But it is not true. Everybody makes mistakes, and everybody deserves love.

Repeat to yourself: "I love myself. I am loveable. I love my life. I love my family."

Avoid thoughts of hate and remove them from your mind as fast as possible. Replace them with thoughts of love.

> *"Every leaf that grows will tell you...*
> *What you sow will bear fruit.*
> *So if you have any sense... my friend*
> *don't plant anything but love."*
>
> -Rumi

Gratitude

When you appreciate life, you are more aware. You are more present in the moment. This acknowledgment makes you happy and feels good. When you are grateful, you take nothing for granted. It is an attitude. Life is a gift; happy people look for what they can be grateful for and what they can be grateful for *now*, instead of thinking about the past or worrying about the future.

When you are grateful, happiness can be felt *now*. When you are grateful, you are focused on what you have, not what you're missing. It brings happiness. As the saying goes, the glass is half-full or half-empty. You appreciate what you have. You may want more, but the more you appreciate what you have and the more grateful you are, the more you get what you want.

I experienced this way of living as a child. When I was a child, I was so grateful for the small things that I had: a toy, eating, playing. I was very happy. I never thought about the things we didn't have or that our neighbor had more than us. When I grew older, I began to think we didn't have enough; I started comparing myself to others instead of being grateful for what I had.

When you have thoughts of gratitude, you cannot have negative thoughts at the same time.

Remember – You Are Not Alone and You Have Support

When you're sick, you need to keep in mind that you're not alone. Feeling lonely is not good for your health. Most of the time, people have the feelings of loneliness rather than really being lonely. Sometimes we need to be proactive and call or talk to our friends and family.

This is part of the action you need to take for your healing. In a Harvard Grant study, the researcher found that one of the main factors of a happy and long life was good, loving relationships, especially if you have somebody who you can trust and rely on.

Feeling that you have other people who support you and you do not have to take care everything by yourself, it makes you more relaxed. A calm mind and body is essential when you are healing. You have many people who will support you such as your family, friends, medical team, and the community.

They are all with you and want to help you. Also remember that there are other patients who have the same illness and are in the process of healing. They may have a better understanding of what you are going through. You can help them and they can help you.

One of the best ways to feel better and have a sense of belonging is to help others, especially patients who have the same illness as you. When you take the focus off yourself and help others, you will heal.

In one example, a few patients who had AIDS were told that they would probably die in a few months. These patients thought, *if we are going to die, why don't we go and help others?* They traveled to Africa and, in the meantime, they got involved in helping others. They took the focus off themselves and put others first.

After several months passed, they were still alive. When they came back and took blood tests, their white blood cell numbers had improved.

Chapter Five
Peaceful Thoughts

"The greatest weapon against stress is our ability

to choose one thought over another."

—William James

Who does not want a serene and peaceful life despite what challenges come to them?

A peaceful mind is a mind that stays in peace under different conditions and stays free of the effect of stress. **Serenity is more precious than gold.** You may ask; is there a magic wand, which we can use to create such a calm mind? Wouldn't it be great if we could have a serene life for as long as we live?

I do not know about such a wand, but I know there are ways for having a peaceful mind and life despite daily stresses. There are techniques that we all can use to keep a calm mind under any condition. The good news is that all these techniques are available to everybody, everywhere, and they are free. Let us learn more about stress and the effects of stress on the body before we talk about how to create a peaceful mind and life.

Stress

What is stress? Scientists describe stress as the outcome of interactions between people and the demands of the environment, especially when we feel the demands exceed our ability to cope. The external forces that cause stress are called *stressors*, and our psychological and biological reaction to that stressor is called the *stress response.*

This response depends on the individual. The same stressor (the same event) will have different meanings for different people, which is why they respond differently. The stressor could be psychological or physical. Psychological stressors include minor issues like traffic conditions or a Christmas gathering, to major ones like divorce or the loss of a child or spouse. Or it could be physical, like a trauma to the body, such as an accident or a physical illness.

In today's society, we talk more about psychological stressors, and they are much more common than physical stressors.

There are two kinds of stress: acute and chronic stress.

Acute stress is typically short-lived, like taking a test or moving to a new place. In acute stress, after it has passed, the body will come back to its normal state. Acute stress increases the sense of judgment and accuracy. Not all stress is bad. Small amounts of stress, such as taking a test or giving a speech, could be good. This kind of stress is good for your brain; it stretches your abilities, and your brain makes new neuronal connections. Small amounts of stress in older people stimulate their brain, mind and increase their cognition.

Chronic stress is prolonged stress that exists for weeks or years. Examples of chronic stress include strained families, failed marriages, and chronic illness, which are continuous and long lasting. Sometimes chronic stresses are as the result of a prolonged series of intermittent events such as difficult encounters at work.

Some people dwell upon past events and continue to have stress even long after the stressful situation has gone. **In these cases, such as resentment, even though the stress is over, the chronic stress is not over.** This is why forgiveness has been emphasized so much. We can't have a peaceful mind and life without forgiveness.

The Stress Response and Its Effect on the Body

The stress response, or fight or flight response, was first described by Dr. Walter B. Cannon. Fight or flight response evolved as a survival mechanism in response to life-threatening situations. Stress response originates in the brain and co-ordinates by the brain. First, the brain perceives the threat which can be unconscious or conscious.

Our perception of threat is affected by our memories, beliefs, and emotions. Different parts and neuronal networks of the brain will be activated during stress response. Then the brain causes activation of two main systems; sympathetic nervous system and the hypothalamus-pituitary-adrenal system. Initially, the sympathetic nervous system will be activated and will cause the release of the hormones noradrenaline and adrenalin.

Then the hypothalamus-pituitary-adrenal system will be activated, causing the release of cortisol. The former system activates first and subsides quickly, whereas the second system starts later and lasts longer. Therefore, we will have increased the stress hormones (mainly noradrenaline, adrenaline and cortisol) during stress response. As the result, the heart rate goes up; muscles become tense and we become ready to act (Fight or flee).

We tend to activate the stress or fight or flight response multiple times a day for stressful situations that are not life threatening. When we are faced with a stressor that could be real or perceived as real, our brain and body prepare with a series of coordinate autonomic, hormonal, immune and behavioral responses. The type, intensity and duration of these responses are depending on the person.

If the intensity and duration of response dropped when it is no longer necessary, this is a successful and normal response. When something is bothering us and makes us, for example, angry, sad or afraid, these are primary emotions and a natural human response. But the problem starts when the response is excessive and abnormal in intensity and duration.

If somebody loses a loved one and becomes sad and shows her sadness by crying, this is a natural and normal emotion. But if the person lets this temporary sadness turn to a long-term sadness and depression, then it becomes harmful to the mind, brain and body.

Repeated stress shuts down activity and reduces volume of the prefrontal cortex (PFC). PFC is the cerebral cortex that covers the front part of the frontal lobe just behind the forehead. PFC is responsible for executive function of the brain, such as decision making, personality expression and moderating social activities and is called CEO of the brain.

PFC, with its connection to amygdala (emotional center of the brain), regulates emotional response. Impairment of PCF regulatory function strengthens amygdala function and causes a vicious cycle of activated stress pathways. The overriding control of the impulse has stopped and may result in unacceptable social behavior.

Stress also impairs higher functions of PFC, such as working memory and attention control. As the result, the response to the stressor changes from a thoughtful and flexible response to an impulsive and habitual response. The stressed person may show inappropriate behavior, which they may regret later on.

Long-term atypical reactions to life stressors may result in different stress-related disorders, from mild to severe, such as PTSD (post-traumatic stress disorder). The stress-related disorders can cause immune dysfunction.

A study has been conducted in Sweden to determine the relationship between stress-related disorders and subsequent autoimmune disease. The study revealed that the patients with stress-related disorders are at increased risks of 41 different autoimmune diseases compared to people without stress-related disorders. The patients with PTSD are at increase risks of multiple autoimmune diseases including rheumatoid arteritis, Crohn's disease and psoriasis.

In chronic stress the stress response is constantly activated and causes harm to the brain and body. Chronic stress has been linked to several emotional and physical illnesses such as depression, high blood pressure and heart disease. Some studies show that many doctor's visits could be due to chronic stress. Stress activates the sympathetic nervous system (a part of the autonomic nervous system) and endocrine system.

One of the main hormones which releases in stress response is cortisol, from the adrenal gland. Cortisol suppresses the immune system and increases the chance of infection and illness. Suppressing the immune system can cause existing tumor cells to grow or develop a new cancer. One study showed that patients with the highest stress were six times more likely to get an infection with cold viruses than those with lesser stress, and they had twice the likelihood of developing symptoms.

In this study, a small amount of flu virus was given to individuals who had maximum and minimal amounts of stress. In these two groups of patients, all other factors were the same.

The long-term fear of cancer may cause further cancer. A study of the patients who lived close to a nuclear reactor showed that they developed more cancer than patients who lived farther away. When studied carefully, the study showed that radiation due to nuclear material was not enough to cause cancer in that area. The cause may have been the impairment of the immune system due to the fear of having cancer that increased the susceptibility to new cancer or promoted the growth of the existing early cancer cells.

The Relaxation Response and Its Effect on the Body

The term relaxation response was initially named by Dr. Herbert Benson. He used this term for physiological changes that happened during meditation. The relaxation response is meant to counter the stress response (fight or flight response). In the relaxation response, the parasympathetic nervous system is activated and calms the body. In this relaxed situation, the blood pressure, heart rate, and acute immune responses all drop.

There are many activities that elicit the relaxation response including: meditation, praying, yoga, gardening, and walking. Regular exercise helps relieve tension.

Exercises such as walking, running, bicycling, yoga, and tai chi elicit the relaxation response.

Regularly engaging in these kinds of activities can help relieve daily stress. You boost relaxation response if, during exercise, you pay attention to being aware of yourself, your feelings, your breathing, and your surroundings. If disruptive thoughts come, gently change them and focus on moving and breathing.

When you walk, pay attention to sights, sounds and smells around you. Notice flowers, leaves, the sun, clouds, fresh air, and bird sounds. These activities quiet the mind and relax the body. They create a state of rest so that healing can take place and the body can repair itself.

You can elicit the relaxation response during daily life, at home and at work. When you get stressed during the day, you should not start feeling bad that you are stressed. Simply take some time for nurturing yourself, you deserve it. When you feel stressed or anxious, find a moment as soon as you can to relax.

Some ways to relax are listening to music, spending a few minutes alone, or taking a walk. These periods of relaxation help you to counteract the toxic effects of stress. The regular practice of these activities illicit the relaxation response and makes your mind quieter. They help you to relieve feeling anxiety and depression. In a simple term, you should try to find some time for relaxing to escape the pressures of daily life.

Sometimes, at work, your boss is demanding something, or at home, your children or spouse are demanding. If you feel stressed, be brave and tell them, "I am feeling stressed and I need take some time off for myself to relax and refresh." In the end, it is good for you *and* them. If you want to have a more profound state of relaxation, you can add methods such as meditation, prayer and yoga to your schedule.

Peace of Mind

Our thoughts in our mind change constantly to demands from the outside world which we receive through our senses and inside world of memories. Our thoughts are also usually associated with feelings and emotions. This information, which is demanding our attention, is always going on inside and around us, making our mind busy and restless.

This is why some people are stressed most of the time and have a hard time staying relaxed. Peace of mind not only associated with our happiness and health, but also it expands to others around us. If each of us has more of a peaceful mind, then we will have a more peaceful family, community and world.

We are responsible for creating our inner peace, and it can be cultivated with various forms of activities such as silence, gardening, and going for a walk. We can also use methods such as Meditation and prayer, which can bring a deeper inner peace.

A Peaceful Mind with Meditation

Meditation is a way to temporarily stop listening to daily life's distractions and listen to the deeper thoughts that come from your unconsciousness. In meditation, the mind is in a deeper, restful state than its usual superficial state that is reacting to different stimuli.

In a meditative state, the mind does not follow the usual stream of thoughts. You go into a deeper state, and the brain waves become slower (alpha waves). By focusing on breathing, you prevent your thoughts from distraction and detach yourself from what is happening in the environment.

There are different ways to meditate. There are many masters and books that they can help you learn how to meditate. The important point is to put some aside time for meditation and relaxation in your schedule. I strongly suggest meditation, especially if you are suffering from anxiety and depression.

Meditation is also important when we are suffering from a physical illness. The disease usually causes fear and stress and meditation would help us to relieve stress and fear and, therefore, our body heals faster.

What Happens During Meditation in the Body?

- Meditation causes physiological and chemical changes in the brain and the body.
- The mind and the body become calmer.

- Because of the activation of the parasympathetic nervous system, the heart, respiratory, and metabolic rate drops.
- In meditation, the stress hormone levels drop and help to normalize the blood pressure.

The benefits of meditation for emotional and physical health have been well documented. Meditation reduces anxiety and panic attacks. Mindfulness meditation can be used for treatment of depression.

A Peaceful Mind through Spirituality

Spirituality has different meanings for different people. Spirituality helps us to slow down and turn inward to our values and beliefs. We choose time for science and stillness.

For some people, spirituality is a connection with a higher power. For other people, spirituality is a sense of having a great purpose or value and connecting to something larger than themselves.

There is convincing evidence throughout history and in different cultures that our bodies will benefit from these spiritual experiences.

Spiritual practices are found in different cultures around the world, and they have some similarities (gathering together to worship, praying, dancing, or mantras). It has been shown that people who have spiritual experiences, such as attending religious services, are happier, have lower blood pressure, and live longer.

After a spiritual gathering, people usually have some degree of internal peace. There are different reasons for the health benefits of spirituality. These include having faith in a higher power; spiritual people may pay more attention to their behavior, and they may have a healthier lifestyle. Being in the spiritual community brings calmness and a feeling of presence. The spiritual practices also give us hope.

Praying has a healing power. All types of prayer help you gain peace of mind, especially the prayer of gratitude, which brings serenity and peace. When you pray and are grateful and do not ask for something, you will find more peace.

Chapter Six
The Effect of Actions on Thoughts

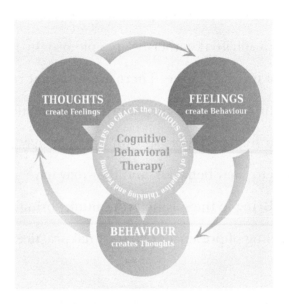

The Effect of Behavior on Thoughts

Your actions trigger thoughts and emotions in your mind. You actually act your way into the feeling which correspond to that action. If you act as if you are already positive and happy, you will feel that way from inside. Your physical state affects your mind and thoughts. The way you sit, stand, and walk affects the way you feel, because these activities affect your thinking. It is called neuro-association. The brain learns to associate certain postures with certain thoughts and feelings. Happy people stand and walk differently from people with depression. Happy people stand straight with their shoulders back.

People with depression bend forward with their head and shoulders down. Not only do your thoughts affect your behavior, but also, your behavior affects your thoughts. Your physiology affects your thinking.

When you have an illness and are in the process of healing, you should act healthy and strong, exercise, take a walk in nature, and get fresh air. These activities affect your brain, your thoughts, and your mind. When you stand tall and straight, your brain has already associated this posture with health and feeling good, and you start feeling better.

You do not have to wait until you feel like it to act in a healthy and happy way. When you act differently, you feel differently. For example, if you merely smile, it activates a series of neuronal networks in your brain that can make you happier. When we act the way we wish to feel, we start feeling that way, and if we repeat an action long enough it will become a habit.

Most of what we think and do daily is habitual. So, for behaving in a certain way, we need to consciously pay attention to what we think. We need to behave in a new way long enough, until this new behavior replaces the old one. Let me first discuss habits, addiction and recovery. I will then talk about some of the daily actions that we can take which make us happier, calmer and healthier.

Habits

A habit will form when a certain neuronal network is activated over and over by repeating a particular task. Every time this particular activity repeats, more and stronger connections are bonded between activated neurons. As this happens unconsciously, you form a habit.

When you repeatedly use the same neurons and their synapses, those neurons and junctions become easier for conducting electrical activity. After forming a habit, similar conditions stimulate the same neurons, and you unconsciously repeat habitual behavior. For example, if you become angry at the certain stimuli over and over again, it uses the same neuronal network, and after some time, it becomes a habit, and you unconsciously become angry whenever those stimuli are present.

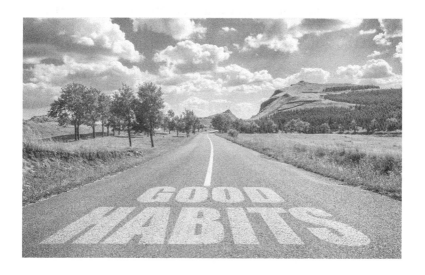

Habits form unconsciously, but if you want to break a habit, it can only be done with conscious effort. Breaking a habit is difficult, but it's possible with effort. We should not repeat routines but replace them with new thoughts and actions. This process needs to be done for a period, usually about two months, until the new habit is formed. For changing a habit, two things need to be done: First, stop doing what you were doing in the past. Second, replace that with a new behavior.

It is difficult to just stop a habit; it is better for it to be replaced with another habit. Then you are using different sets of neurons in the response to the same stimuli. For example, if you get upset and scream because of traffic, and if you wanted to change this habit, the next time you're in traffic, you shouldn't scream. Instead, do something different. For example, say, "I am calm." You basically start using new sets of neurons.

Changing habits takes time, and persistence is essential. There are three steps to changing a habit:

1. The first step is recognizing that a certain habit is not useful and deciding you really want to change it.

2. The second step is no longer having that undesirable thought or action.

3. The third step is replacing it with a new thought and action and committing to do it for at least two months.

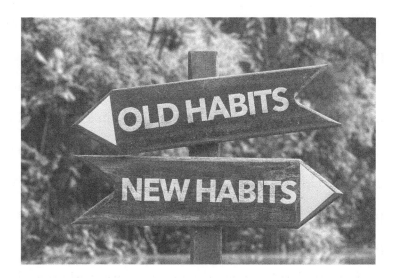

Addiction and the Immature Brain of an Adolescent

The development and maturation of the human brain is parallel to the evolution of the brain. The neocortex (the newer part of the brain) develops last, and some areas may take up to twenty years to mature. Therefore, adolescents have more risk for addiction than older adults.

Some drugs form habits with a powerful influence on the brain, especially the networks associated with reward. Its influence becomes so powerful that it overcomes the rational brain. Addiction is associated with the reward network; some drugs cause the release of dopamine in the nucleus accumbens (a region associated with rewards and pleasurable sensations).

Addiction uses the same pathway and the same neurotransmitter (dopamine) that we use in learning. The drug causes the release of so much more dopamine that can't be released with usual fun activities. Therefore, the person goes back to using drugs to give him/her the same pleasure that got from the previous use.

Repeated substance use permanently reshapes the pathways in the brain. Because the adolescent brain has not fully developed, there is more of a chance that they will become addicted. The earlier someone starts using drugs, the higher chance they end up with a bigger problem.

Scientifically, there is no safe age for drinking; there is no valid evidence that the brain has matured by age twenty-one.

When you initially use alcohol or drugs, you may say, "Oh, it's not me; I will not become addicted."

But sometime later, you're not able to control yourself because of the pathway that is created in the brain through using the substance over and over. The pleasure of getting that drug becomes more powerful than the consequences of using the drug.

The brain does something to achieve pleasure or avoid pain. For an addicted person, at some point, this desire for pleasure becomes so strong that he/she may sacrifice the most valuable things, such as health and family, to receive the drug.

Therefore, what a child and adolescent do daily is more crucial than an adult. At this age the rational part of the brain has not developed yet and they act based on their emotions. They do what brings them pleasure without thinking about the negative consequences later on. Their brain also has more plasticity and they learn it faster, and the structure of the brain will change, therefore, it will be more difficult to change this behavior later on.

Addiction is treatable and complete remission is possible. However, it could be a long process and multiple efforts may be needed. The relapse is part of the process, because the brain physically needs to change and start using new neuronal networks. The addicted individuals, their family and treating team should have hope and persistence. A good treatment usually includes different components, such as the mental health facility and family. A good treatment regularly monitors the progress of the patient and adjusts accordingly.

We Must Practice the Person We Wish to Be.

"Act the way you'd like to be and soon you'll be the way you act."

- Leonard Cohen

Every day, from the time we wake up until we sleep again, the way we speak and act affect our thoughts and feelings. We can choose how we are going to behave despite the different situations and how we feel. If our beliefs, thoughts and behavior harmonize together, we will live the life we truly want. Some activities that we can do every day to have a happy, calm and healthy day are as followed:

- **Falling asleep and waking up**

What you think about the last five minutes before you fall asleep is very important. During the night when you are asleep, those thoughts will process unconsciously. If you have negative thoughts or emotions, try to change them before falling asleep.

For example, if you have a fear of a medical test or its outcome, try somehow to change your state of mind to a happy, calm, and hopeful state before falling asleep. You can turn on the light and read an inspiring book or pray.

Do not sleep with thoughts of fear, anxiety, and worry. Try to calm down before you fall asleep.

When you wake up in the morning, try to start the day with positive thoughts and good feelings. Take a few minutes to reflect on the aspects of your life that you are grateful for, feeling love by recalling the people you love, or praying and/or meditating. These practices put you in a good tone for the whole day.

- **Speak only health and healing**

  "Never affirm or repeat about your health
  what you do not wish to be true."
  —Ralph Waldo Trine

Say the things that you want to happen to you, not the things you fear or don't want. You say your vision and what you want to happen, not the present circumstances. You need to talk positively, especially when you have an illness.

Even though all the circumstances around you may indicate you are weak, you are sick, or that you may die. You need to say and believe the opposite. You need to say what you want to happen. Say, "I am strong, I am well, and I will live."

Do not own the disease; keep yourself detached from it. For example, you can say, "This illness is bothering me," or "I am suffering from this illness." Watch your words; talk about your illness in a positive way. If people ask you how you're doing, say, "I am improving, and I will defeat this disease."

When you find the smallest improvement, be grateful, celebrate it, and talk about it: "Today my test was a little better; today my temperature was better, and I am feeling better."

Speak as if you are already healed, and repeat to yourself, "I am healed," or "I am healing."

As soon as negative words come to your mouth, change them to positive ones or don't say anything at all.

As Joel Osteen said, *"You make your world with your words."*

When you speak your thoughts, they come closer to reality. Say positive words about your healing, even if you don't feel like it. When you want to complain, it's better to stop and say something positive. When you say positive words, it affects your thoughts. You'll feel better and heal faster.

- **Incantation/affirmation**

Autosuggestion is very powerful. It's very important that you suggest to your brain what you want. Every moment you have a chance, you should repeat some positive phrases that inspire you. Say these positive phrases out loud or under your breath. Repeat these affirmations and inspiring words thousands of times a day, at every chance you can.

It could be at home, waiting in the doctor's office, or driving; say positive and inspiring words. Say affirmations such as: "I am getting better every day in every way," or simply, "I feel good (even if you don't), I am healed, I am healing."

• **Play and laughter**

Sir William Osler called laughter, *"the music of life."* Laughter and humor make it easier to tolerate and handle difficult situations. A study has shown that patients with humor recover better than patients who rarely laugh.

• **Writing your progress**

Writing and journaling during the healing process helps in many ways. Writing causes you to remember better. Buy a nice journal with a happy and calming design, one that inspires you. Write all the positive and uplifting information that you know about your progress. Write about the good results that are happening and those you want to happen. Read them during the day, especially in the morning after waking up and in the evening before falling asleep.

Write your vision; specify what you want to happen. This process of writing will reduce your stress. It consolidates the memory and gives you clarity of thinking. Writing activates the basal ganglia and frontal lobe; you'll see your situation with less confusion.

- **Vision board**

Prepare a vision board and put on it what you love and want to happen. Put it somewhere so you can see it frequently. Put pictures, writing, and future goals on it. Sit in front of it, relax, visualize your goals, and let them sink into your unconscious mind.

Chapter Seven
Put It All Together for a
Happy and Healthy Life

*"Act is the blossom of thought, and joy and suffering
are its fruits; thus a man garner in the sweet
and bitter fruitage of his own husbandry."*

—James Allen

Healthy Lifestyle

Nothing is more valuable than our health. All other important things in our life depend on our health. Our health is our responsibility and our healing starts with us. Our body has multiple systems that work constantly to keep us healthy. If something happens to our body, it will start the healing process right away.

We can help our body to keep our health or lose it with our behavior, for keeping our health comes responsibility. Fortunately, there are only a few essential factors and we are all capable of doing them. The essential factors include: healthy eating, regular physical activity, and proper sleep, avoid smoking and drugs, excessive alcohol, and dangerous behaviors such as fast driving.

Of course, positive thinking, optimism and a peaceful mind, as I explained in detail in chapter 4 and 5, are essential in emotional and physical health. Our healthy behavior is important and can affect the body at the level of gene expression. A person may have a gene for a specific disease, but with healthy behavior this person may go through their whole life without getting that disease. But if we ignore any of these factors, our health will be negatively affected.

Our body has a self-healing system. We should try to help and not interfere with this self-healing process. Many emergency room and doctor visits are due to our own unhealthy choices and harmful habits. A lot of diseases such as diabetes, high blood pressure, and ulcers can be prevented or improved with a proper, healthy lifestyle. I have seen patients with different infections. Most of these infections could be prevented with some percussion.

Following a few, simple steps daily can help you enjoy a healthy and happy life and prevent you from pain and suffering later on.

Medicine

You should take advantage of all modern medical and surgical treatment. See your doctor regularly and take her or his advice. Traditional medicine has progressed significantly in different areas. We are able to diagnose and treat diseases faster and better. This needs to be taken advantage of and used.

I see many patients with severe head injuries after trauma. They need supportive treatment in intensive care units. Sometimes, they need surgery; they need medication, and they need care. Without these medical and surgical treatments, the patients could lose their lives.

You should have regular checkups with your doctor. It is best to prevent a disease, but if that is not the case then it is best to diagnose the disease as soon as possible. The sooner the diagnosis, the easier and faster the treatment and healing would begin. Do not postpone the necessary treatment.

If you need to get more information or another opinion, please do so. It is natural to be scared after hearing that you have an illness, but despite these fears, we need the find the best treatment and take care of it. Most of illnesses today have treatment options that will help you heal. When you are sick, your most important job in your life is to get the proper treatment and become healthy again.

This attitude is important for illnesses such as diabetes and high blood pressure, because Pain is not typically associated with them. These patients have a tendency to ignore the symptoms and unfortunately the complications can arise. I have seen many patients with brain bleeding due to uncontrolled high blood pressure.

If you are sick, go to see your physician or go to the hospital or emergency department. You should go with hope and the attitude that "with the help of the medical team, I will get rid of this disease and return to my natural state of health."

Why did I add the section of healthy life style and medicine to this book that is about using your thoughts to heal? Because I want be clear, when I am saying use your thoughts to heal, it does not mean to ignore the healthy life style, prevention, traditional medical and surgical treatment. When you are positive, happy, hopeful and calm, you will heal faster when you are getting your treatment. During the treatment process, you will have more energy, stamina and persistence.

I also should add we should use any kind of treatment available that can help us. There are multiple modalities for treatment, that's why it is called "the art of medicine". We need to check to be sure the suggested treatment technique is real, proven, scientific and makes sense.

I have known of some people who put their treatment in the hands of some random healers and unfortunately, they did not heal or lost their lives. We also need to remember that not all treatments work on everybody the same. One kind of treatment may work for one person, and not for another.

Find Out if There is Contributing Factor to Your Illness

In order to optimally prevent and treat disease, you must address the possible mental and emotional causes that make you susceptible to illness. For example:

- Do you have a problem in your relationship that is bothering you?
- Do you have a purpose in your life that make you want to live and achieve it?
- Are you depressed or stressed?
- Are you enjoying your work?
- Do you have resentment from the past that needs to be resolved?

If any of these conditions may have been involved in getting the disease; you should try your best to eliminate them. Otherwise, after treating the disease, it may return. I have seen many patients with a negative mental state return to the hospital over and over. If something is going on in our life that make us uneasy and/or brings us down, we need to think and find a way to solve it.

Depending on the situation, different actions may need to be taken. There is always a way. You can't afford to tolerate something that you do not like for a long time. It will cost you your mental, emotional and physical health. It may not be anybody's fault. The problems will not be solved with blaming and lots of time, no one or situation should be blamed.

In my own life, it took me a long time to realize that the person that needs to change is me. Because of my old beliefs and habits, I was just not able to see the situation clearly. I created a lot of problems and stress for myself, until I became aware and started changing my thoughts, old beliefs and habits. It did take a lot of time and energy and I am still working on it. But I tell you, it is worth every minute of it, my life is much happier and calmer.

Accept Yourself as You Are

Becoming aware and accepting our weaknesses and imperfections is the key to realizing our true strength. Then, by facing these weaknesses, such as bad habits, we discover and experience a feeling of well-being and that we can overcome our problems. We start changing daily and become wiser and start seeing our potential. You must remember, there should not be any guilt or judgment toward yourself if you have any disturbing emotion. Some people may feel ashamed that they have some emotional problems like depression.

Emotional and psychological problems are as real and important as physical diseases, and you need to get proper help to heal. It is not your fault that you got sick; there are multiple factors involved in any disease. Even if you had some unhealthy behavior in the past, it is in the past; judging yourself and feeling guilty are negative feelings, they will affect you negatively.

You really should not feel bad if you had a negative thought; you just need to replace it with a positive one.

Simply, you observe your thoughts and change them to positive thoughts. Especially in the time of disease, you may have negative thoughts and fears; these are all natural.

Be kind to yourself; love and accept yourself for who you are and with all your habits, even if you wish to change some of them. When you love yourself, it's not only a very positive feeling that affects your healing, you also will have more energy and stamina.

Accepting oneself is important for having a healthy and clear mind. When you accept yourself as you are, you stop fighting with yourself. Instead, you know yourself better. You know and accept your strength and weaknesses, and now you know where you are. When you accept yourself, it will become easier to be positive, happy and calm, which are very important for your health. Then you think about your goals, visualize them and make a plan to achieve them. You may need to change some old habits with new ones, and sometimes it is difficult, but if you keep persisting, you will achieve your goal.

Do not engage in negative self-talk. For example, you may have done so many good things during the day, but you did one thing that you did not like. Your thoughts may go over and over it with negative emotions. Replace this instead with loving and kind feelings toward yourself. I sometimes hear people say, "I am a bad person." This is one of the worst things you can tell yourself.

You simply made a mistake; next time, you will make a different decision and choose differently. You learn from it and let it go. Forgive yourself. During your lifetime, you will become ill, physically or emotionally. Your thoughts not only affect your susceptibility to illnesses, they also may affect the nature and timing of your death.

It has been shown that for people who live a long life, the special qualities that stand out (besides exercise and proper diet) are happiness, peacefulness, and being easy on themselves (being at ease and relaxed).

Practice What You Know Now

You have read how important your thoughts are for happiness, health, and healing. You need to practice them until they become effortless and become your habit.

Take responsibility for your thoughts and what you are thinking, and take the proper action. Every day practice the following:

- **Think positively**

  If you have negative thoughts and beliefs about your health and healing, change them to positive ones as fast as you can. When negative thoughts come to your mind, say "Cancel," and replace them with positive thoughts.

- **Be happy.** Make an effort every day to increase your happiness and, with that, not only will you be joyful, but you will also be healthier. Say, "I want to feel good."

- **Be hopeful.** Become an optimist and prepare for the best, not for the worst. If the worst comes up, you will take care of it.

- **Stay calm.** You will likely experience stress every day in your life, especially when you have a disease. Find the best way to cope; regulate your stress response and how much it will affect your health. Find a way to be more relaxed; pay attention to other things that calm you down and elicit the relaxation response.

Be relaxed and do whatever you can to stay in a state of peacefulness. Healing takes place in the state of relaxation. Your health and healing depend on it.

- **Speak only happiness, health, and healing**

    Talk about the good things happening in your life.

    Be happy for other people's happiness.

"There is power in words; what you say is what you get."

—Zig Ziglar

Train Your Brain in the Direction of Happiness, Calmness and Health

During the thought process you will have a series of electrical and chemical activities in certain neuronal networks in your brain. The changes in the brain initially are temporary, and after you change your thoughts, the electrical and chemical activities disappear.

But if thoughts are repeated, the structural changes will happen and the brain will rewire. Then you start thinking, responding and behaving differently. Because your brain has rewired, it is not going to be easy and comfortable to think and behave like before. You become more comfortable behaving in the new way that has become your habit.

It is very important what you think and do today, because it is not only changing your body and outside world, but also, it will change your brain. These changes in your brain increase the chance of you thinking and acting the same tomorrow and in the future. The happier you are today, there is a good chance you will be happier tomorrow.

The set point of happiness or calmness is your base line happiness and calmness in the usual circumstances. If you have a higher set point of happiness or calmness, even if you have a difficulty or a stressful situation, you are going to be happier and calmer compared to somebody with a lower set point.

The practices such as meditation, praying, yoga, and walking in nature bring up the set point of calmness and peace of mind. You basically become a calmer person. If someone has a higher set point of happiness, they will be even happier in a joyful event compared to somebody with the lower set point.

The point is, the happier and calmer your thoughts are, the happier and calmer your life is. When you make your daily schedule, do not forget to put several few minutes of interval for your joy and peace of mind time. These joy and peace of mind times not only helps you to keep your joy and calmness in your daily work, but also, they keep your brain and mind healthy.

Train your brain to stay positive until it becomes your default. Serious disease can cause depression and anxiety if we let them. You need to actively think positively and stay happy, optimistic, and peaceful. Repeating positive thoughts gradually shifts your beliefs, and they become part of your unconscious mind. Then the positive thoughts and beliefs will work, even in your sleep.

Every time you train your brain to think positively, it becomes easier and easier, and you become more and more positive.

Certain people always seem to be up; they are always happy and joyful. When you check with them, they also have problems. Happy people do have problems and challenges, but they find a way to deal with them.

It is very important that people with illnesses feel good; those around them should encourage them to feel good.

Surround yourself with happy people.

You may say, "I have a problem with my health; I have pain." I agree; you have a problem. But when you feel good, you take the depression and stress off. You will be happier and calmer, and you'll also heal faster. You'll start coming from the mental state of, *I am powerful; I can do it.* In this state of mind, you'll find a solution.

Persist (Never Quit)

"You will succeed if you persevere; and you will find a joy in overcoming obstacles."

-Helen Keller

You do not know the future. At any moment, circumstances may change. But you must keep going. First of all, you need to practice positive thinking for some time until these thoughts become part of your subconscious mind and become beliefs and habits.

Depending on the belief and habit, it may take 66 days, or up to 6 months. Basically, the structure of the network related to those beliefs and habits needs to change. Some of the connections must be disabled and new connections must be made. It does take time, because when you think differently, it will affect the DNA of the active neurons and make new proteins and new connections. This process takes time and needs patience.

The healing process takes time. The time for the healing of different organs in the body varies. The skin heals in a few days, but the bone heals over a few weeks. Treating some of the diseases may require medication for a specific time. For example, treating a bone infection, you may need intravenous antibiotics for 3 months.

Some of the diseases may need staged surgery or a combination of surgery, radiation and chemotherapy. I tell my patients, this is the time you need to think positively, be happy, be hopeful and have faith. It is easy to have faith when everything going well. But the real test of faith comes when a person is diagnosed with serious illness. It is not easy, but this is the time, do not let fear take over.

This is the time to have faith. This is the time to stay calm. This is the time to stay happy and positive. This is the time to believe that you are going to heal. This is like the time you are in the storm. If you keep steady, eventually, the storm will pass. It is very important that you keep going and do not get tired or disappointed. In any survival situation, the people who survived are the ones who kept going because they were committed to the end result.

"It matters if you just don't give up."
—Stephen Hawking

All your actions produce results if you are patient and keep doing the right things. Eventually, they produce good results. Persistence is essential for healing in stroke and trauma patients. Rehabilitation is the key for treatment in these groups of patients. They need to persist and continue to take the necessary steps to heal.

I've seen many patients following a stroke, head injury, and paralysis. The patients, who kept a good attitude, hope and continued doing whatever they needed to do have the best results. You basically keep your vision of what you want to happen and keep going towards that vision. You need to have a healing goal and you will not stop until you get there, it does not matter how difficult and how long is going to take.

I believe, if you have a serious illness, you should not ask the doctors how long you are going to live. The Doctors give you an average number based on some studies, which may not even be accurate. But whatever it is, you do not need to know or believe in it. You should believe that "I am going to heal" and go do your best and get any kind of treatment which is available.

I would not tell any patient how long they are going to live. There are so many factors and patients are different. I also think this kind of news is depressing and frightening and only adds to the patient's stress. If you believe their time limit accuracy, the brain and body respond to this accordingly and may start shutting down.

I strongly suggest ignoring this kind of news and instead, believing exactly the opposite. I believe until the last moment that we are on this Earth that we should have hopes, goals, and plans for the future. This kind of attitude is good for our family as well. I want to see my family members happy, calm and full of hope and faith, not fear and hopelessness even when they pass away.

Our life is a gift and we should enjoy every moment of it, as much as we can. We may have challenges; we will work it out somehow. Tony Robbins said, *"If you are committed, you will find a way."* Your Life is a journey and you should go out there and find a way. Do not stay at home and have a self-pity party; start working on your healing right away.

The struggling, temporarily getting sad and afraid, getting treatment such as surgery, medication, even radiation and chemotherapy are part of this journey. **Who said you should be depressed and anxious when you are having radiation and chemotherapy? Why not be happy, calm and have hope and love while having the treatment?** I have no doubt that results are going to better. Norman Vincent Peale said, *"It is always too early to quit."*

You Have Control over Your Happiness, Health, and Healing

Having feelings of control in your health and healing, a feeling that you can do something about it is crucial. Thoughts of doubt and fear accomplish nothing. As long as your brain is alive and your mind is working, you are the master. Of course, you need to get medical help, advice, and surgery, (if needed) but you have autonomy; you are in charge.

You need to do whatever is necessary for your healing. The amazing part about it is that you do have control over your health and healing. When you feel you are in control, you do your best; it's easier for your body to return to its usual state of health. When you feel in control, you feel responsible; you participate and do whatever is necessary. You do not bring excuses or feel self-pity or depression.

Thoughts and feelings of being in control will help you stay in peace. Remember you are always the master of your life, even in your weakest state.

The Future Mind, Brain and Body Connection

The mind and brain are greatest mysteries in all of nature. Our knowledge of the brain and mind has been transformed by advances in neuroscience and technology, such as different types of brain MRI (magnetic resonance imaging) and other brain scans. There are advances in neuroscience for treating mental illness and dementia.

Medical science has advanced rapidly for prevention and treatment of different diseases. For example, the Human Genome project (HGP) changed the scientific and medical landscape. The resources created with HGP, help to detect the genetic predisposition to some diseases, improve the diagnosis and treatment of diseases.

We are learning more about the mind from studying the biology of the brain. There are several projects focusing on the neuronal circuits of the brain. The researcher able to track the activity patterns in brain cells after we have an experience or a thought; these studies lead us to understand how the brain operates.

With all these advances, we understand better how our thoughts and feeling affect our bodies.

Keep learning about different ideas and get out of your comfort zone, it will change and expand your mind. You become more aware and you see the reality better. You become more open minded. Ignorance is one of the greatest enemies of the human being.

Keep learning more about your brain, thoughts and mind and how they affect your happiness, peace of mind, health and healing. Everybody needs to know more about them. It does not matter what age, or what kind of job you are doing. Everybody wants to be happy, calm and healthy.

If these three (health, happiness and calmness) are missing from our life, we can't have a fulfilled life. Most of us, during our lifetime, will have some kind of emotional or physical illness. When you know that you can use your thoughts to heal, it will give you hope and power. Your healing process starts with you. Do not wait for someone to heal you.

You start doing what you can do and of course, get necessary help from professionals. The more you know about it and the more techniques you learn, the better you'll understand it, and the better you'll do it. You can learn more by reading books, listening to tapes, or going to seminars, as well as learn from people who are happy, peaceful, healed and healing. Do not forget to help other people to be happier and heal. When you do that, you will be happier and heal yourself.

Thank you for choosing and reading this book. I hope it helps you with your happiness, health and healing.

"Strive to live fully until the last moment you have. This attitude gives you hope, energy, and liveliness. You will live like a hero."

-Mahmoud Rashidi

"Your illness does not define you; your strength and courage do."

—Unknown

"Live with Passion"

-Tony Robbins

Glossary

- Acetylcholine: A transmitter at the neuromuscular junction that causes muscle to contract. It also can be found in the brain.

- Alpha waves: Brain waves at the time of relaxation, such as meditation.

- Alzheimer's disease: The most common form of dementia, caused by accumulation of tangles inside nerve cells and progressing to nerve cell death.

- Amygdala: An almond-shaped structure deep in the medial temporal lobe and is a component of the limbic system. It is a center for emotion and emotional behaviors, especially fear.

- Autonomic nervous system: The part of the nervous system that largely acts unconsciously and controls the internal organs like the heart and digestive system. It has two main divisions: sympathetic and parasympathetic nervous systems.

- Axon: A nerve fiber that transmits electrical impulses away from nerve cells.

- Basal ganglia: Large subcortical nuclear masses that consist of the caudate nucleus, putamen, and globus pallidus and are associated with many functions, including voluntary motor control and coordination.

- Beta waves: Brain waves at time of high brain activity, like problem solving.

- Brain death: When the brain irreversibly loses its electrochemical activity and function.

- Central nervous system: system of the organs in the body, Including the brain and spinal cord.

- Cerebellum: *Cerebellum* means "little brain." It is the most posterior part of the brain, located behind the upper part of the brainstem. Its function includes movement coordination, balance, and equilibrium.

- Cerebral cortex: The external layer of the brain. It is the center for higher functions: thinking, imagination, creativity, decision, and so on.

- Concussion: A concussion is a temporary loss of brain function. People with concussion after a mild head injury have reversible chemical changes in their brains.

- Consciousness: The state of awareness of ourselves, our thoughts, our feelings, and our surroundings.

- Corpus callosum: The largest bundle of nerve fibers (about two hundred million) in the brain that connect the right and left hemisphere of the brain together and allow communication between them.

- Cortisol: A hormone released from the adrenal gland in response to stress.

- Cranial nerves: Nerve fibers that directly connect to the brain through the opening in the cranium and carry nerve impulses to and from the brain.

- Cranium: The cranium is the part of the skull that covers and protects the brain (the skull includes the cranium and mandible).

- Delta waves: Brain waves during sleep.

- Dementia: The decline of memory and other thinking skills that interfere with daily life activities.

- Dendrites: Dendrites are short nerve fibers that carry information from other neurons to the nerve cell body.

- DNA: Deoxyribonucleic acid is a molecule in the cell nucleus that carries gene instructions.

- EEG: Electroencephalogram is an electrophysiological monitoring of the brain's electrical activities.

- Emotion: A mental state with feeling associated with change in a person's physiology and behavior. There are six primary emotions: fear, anger, joy, sadness, disgust, and surprise.

- Free radicals: Any atom or molecule with a single unpaired electron that seeks to become paired with other electrons and make other molecule unstable. It causes damage to DNA, protein, and cells.

- GABA: Gamma aminobutyric acid is the main inhibitory neurotransmitter in the central nervous system.

- Gene: A region of DNA, the basic physical and functional unit of heredity.

- Hippocampus: A horseshoe-shaped subcortical structure that belongs to the limbic system. It is important in consolidation of short-term memory to long-term memory.

- Hypothalamus: A region of the brain located under the thalamus. It forms the floor and wall of the third ventricle. It connects the nervous system to the endocrine system via the pituitary gland and controls many physiological functions, including thermal regulation, thirst, hunger, and sleep.

- Limbic system: A collection of structures including the amygdala, hypothalamus, and hippocampus. The limbic system has a variety of functions, including emotions and long-term memory.

- Mirror neuron: A neuron that fires when we act or observe the same action performed by someone else. Mirror neurons are important in developing empathy, understanding others, and learning by imitating others.

- Myelin sheath: A fatty tissue that wraps around some of the axons and works as insulation. It increases the speed of the transmission of nerve impulses and is essential for proper function of the nervous system.

- Neuroglia: Glial cells that support neurons.

- Neuron: Nerve cell that generates and transmits nerve impulses.

- Neurotransmitter: A chemical messenger that transmits signals across the synapse between neurons or a neuron and target cell.

- Nucleus accumbens: Part of the basal forebrain. It has a central role in reward and feeling of pleasure.

- Parasympathetic nervous system: The division of the autonomic nervous system that relaxes the body. When activated, it lowers the blood pressure, heart rate, and respiratory rate.

- Peripheral nervous system: The sensory and motor neurons outside the brain and spinal cord.

- Plasticity: The ability of the brain to change and rewire at any age.

- Prefrontal cortex: Part of the brain that is located in front of the frontal lobe. It is responsible for many complex behaviors like rational thinking, reasoning, planning, and judgment.
- Serotonin: A neurotransmitter that has an important role in feeling happy.
- Sympathetic nervous system: Part of the autonomic nervous system that is activated in response to threats and is responsible for the fight-or-flight response.
- Synapse: Tiny gap between nerve fibers or between nerve fiber and the target cell that permit electrical or chemical signals to pass from neurons to other neurons or to receptor cells.
- Theta waves: Brain waves during daydreaming and sleep.

Unconscious: The part of the mind that can't be accessed by conscious mind.

Bibliography

Allen F. Harrison and Robert M. Bramson. *The Art of Thinking: The Classic Guide to Increasing Brain Power.* The Berkley Publishing Group, 2002.

Andrea Nani and Andrea E. Cavanna. *Brain, Consciousness, and Causality.* Cambridge, MA: Cosmology Science Publishers, 2011.

Anna Wise. *Awakening the Mind: A Guide to Mastering the Power of Your Brain Waves.* Jeremy P. Tarcher/Penguin, 2002.

Bernie S. Siegel. *Love, Medicine & Miracles.* MJF Books, 2011.

Bruce Lipton. *The Biology of Belief: Unleashing the Power of Consciousness, Matter & Miracles.* Carlsbad, CA: Hay House, 2011.

Bryan Kolb. *Brain Plasticity and Behavior.* Lawrence Erlbaum Associates, Inc., 1995.

Caroline Leaf. *Switch on Your Brain: The Key to Peak Happiness, Thinking, and Health*. Baker Books, 2015.

Catherine Collin. *The Psychology Book: Big Ideas Simply Explained*. DK Publishing, 2012.

Charles Duhigg. *The Power of Habit: Why We Do What We Do in Life and Business*. Random House Trade Paperbacks, 2014.

Daniel Bor and others. *New Scientist INSTANT EXPERT: How Your Brain Works*. Nicholas Brealey Publishing, 2017

Deepak Chopra, M.D. *QUNATUM HEALING: EXPLORING THE FRONTIERS OF MIND/BODY MEDICINE*. Batman Book, 1990

Doc Childre, Howard Martin, and Donna Beech. *The Heartmath Solution*. HarperCollins, 1999.

Ellen Langer. "A Mindful Alternative to the Mind/Body Problem." *Journal of Cosmology*, 14, 2011.

Henri Cohen and Brigitte Stemmer. *Consciousness and Cognition: Fragments of Mind and Brain*. Elsevier Ltd., 2007.

James Allen. *As a Man Thinketh*. John F. Blair, 2010.

Jeffrey Mishlove. *Roots of Consciousness: The Classic Encyclopedia of Consciousness Studies Revised and Expanded.* Council Oak Books, 1993.

John B. Arden. *Rewire Your Brain; Think Your Way to a Better Life.* Hoboken, NJ: John Wiley & Sons, Inc., 2010.

Jonah Lehrer. *How We Decide.* Houghton Mifflin Harcourt, 2009.

Joseph T. Hallinan. *Why We Make Mistakes.* BROADWAY BOOKS, 2009.

Joseph Murphy. *The Power of Your Subconscious Mind.* Penguin Books, 2008.

Eric R. Kandel, James H. Schwartz, and Thomas M. Jessell. *Principles of Neural Science,* Fourth Edition. McGraw-Hill, 2000.

L. Dossey, et al. "Consciousness: What is it?" *Journal of Cosmology,* 14, 2011.

Lisa Rankin. *Mind over Medicine: Scientific Proof That You Can Heal Yourself.* Hay House, 2013.

Malcolm B. Carpenter. *Core Text of Neuroanatomy,* Fourth Edition. Williams & Wilkins, 1996.

Michael S. Sweeney. *Brain: The Complete Mind: How It Develops, How It Works, and How to Keep It Sharp.* National Geographic Society, 2014.

Michio Kaku. *THE FUTURE OF THE MIND.* Anchor Books, 2015

Norman Doidge. *The Brain that Changes Itself; Stories of Personal Triumph from the Frontiers of Brain Science.* Penguin Books. 2007.

Paul David Nussbaum. *Save Your Brain: 5 Things You Must Do to Keep Your Mind Young and Sharp.* McGraw-Hill Professional, 2010.

Paul Martin. *The Healing Mind: The Vital Links between Brain and Behavior, Immunity and Disease.* St. Martin's Press, 1999.

Pierce J. Howard. *The Owner's Manual for the Brain: The Ultimate Guide to Peak Mental Performance at All Ages.* HarperCollins, 2014.

Rhawn Joseph. "Origins of Thought: Consciousness, Language, Egocentric Speech and the Multiplicity of Mind." *Journal of Cosmology,* 14, 2011.

Roger Penrose and Stuart Hameroff. "Consciousness in the Universe: Neuroscience, Quantum Space-Time Geometry, and Orch OR Theory." *Journal of Cosmology,* 14, 2011.

Ronald Potter–Efron. *Healing the Angry Brain.* MJF Books, 2012.

Sharon Begley. *Train Your Mind, Change Your Brain.* Ballantine Books, 2007.

Tony Wright and Graham Gynn. *Return to the Brain of Eden: Restoring the Connection between Neurochemistry and Consciousness.* Simon and Schuster, 2014.

William James. *The Stream of Consciousness.* First published in *Psychology,* 1892, *Journal of Cosmology,* 14, 2011.

William James. *The Stream of Thoughts.* First published in *The Principles of Psychology,* 1890, *Journal of Cosmology,* 14, 2011.

Index

H

Habit 9, 15, 27, 55, 58, 59, 72,
92, 132, 133, 134, 135,
145, 150, 151, 152, 153,
156, 158, 176

Habitual 9, 14, 77, 121, 132, 133

Happiness xi, xiii, xiv, xv, xvii,
xix, 9, 41, 62, 75, 76, 87,
88, 89, 90, 91, 92, 94, 99,
102, 107, 109, 112, 126,
153, 154, 155, 156, 162,
164, 165, 176

Harvard xxii, 94, 102, 113

Healed xii, 95, 105, 108, 140,
141, 165

Healing xi, xii, xiii, xiv, xv, xvii,
xxviii, 9, 52, 55, 62, 72, 73,
74, 75, 76, 81, 83, 84, 85,
86, 98, 102, 105, 110, 111,
113, 114, 124, 129, 131,
139, 140, 141, 142, 144,
145, 147, 152, 153, 154,
155, 159, 160, 162, 163,
165, 166, 176, 178, 179

Health xi, xii, xiv, xv, xvii, xviii,
8, 9, 19, 20, 21, 26, 35, 36,
45, 46, 47, 48, 49, 50, 51,
52, 55, 57, 58, 62, 73, 74,
75, 76, 81, 82, 83, 84, 85,
86, 90, 91, 94, 95, 113,
126, 128, 129, 131, 137,
138, 139, 144, 145, 148,
150, 152, 153, 154, 155,
158, 162, 163, 165, 176

Healthy xi, xiv, xv, xxii, 19, 21,
27, 32, 33, 34, 35, 37, 39,
44, 50, 51, 52, 61, 72, 74,
76, 77, 81, 82, 83, 95, 102,
106, 107, 108, 131, 138,
144, 145, 146, 147, 148,
152, 157, 165

Hear xxvi, 5, 86, 103, 107, 152

Heart 19, 22, 34, 35, 61, 63, 64,
65, 66, 89, 94, 119, 122,
123, 128, 167, 172

Heartbeat 14

Helplessness 96, 104

Hemisphere 22, 23, 30, 169

Heroin 40

108, 109, 110, 113, 137,
139, 140, 149, 151, 152,
153, 154

Neocortex 135

Nerve xxiv, 23, 25, 26, 28, 31,
44, 64, 109, 167, 168, 169,
170, 172, 173

Nervous system 53, 56, 62, 63,
64, 65, 66, 67, 69, 82, 118,
119, 122, 123, 128, 167,
168, 170, 171, 172, 173

Network 3, 4, 6, 11, 30, 50, 54,
56, 71, 73, 87, 107, 118,
131, 132, 133, 135, 137,
155, 158

Neurochemical 48

Neurodegenerative 40, 49

Neurogenesis 42

Neuroglia 25, 172

Neuron 2, 3, 5, 10, 13, 23, 25,
26, 28, 30, 31, 32, 33, 37,
41, 42, 44, 47, 48, 55, 56,
105, 107, 132, 134, 159,
170, 171, 172, 173

Neuroscience xiii, xiv, xvii,
xviii, 9, 88, 163, 179

Neuroscientists 17, 55

Neurosurgery xi, xii, xxiii,
xxvii, xxviii

Neurotransmitter 26, 27, 38,
41, 88, 93, 100, 136, 170,
172, 173

Noble xxii

Norepinephrine 26, 41, 93

Normal 3, 117, 119, 120

Nuclear 122, 123, 168

Nucleus accumbens 88,
136, 172

Nutrition 34

Nuts 38, 39

O

Observer 48, 98

Occipital 23

Olfactory 48

Omega 37, 99

Opioid 40

Optimism xiii, xv, 102, 145

T